HOW TO HAVE FUN WITH YOUR BODY

By MICHAEL LESTER

Original Idea and Title:
SUSAN SUBTLE
Design and Art Direction:
KATE GODFREY
Photography:
MIKKEL AALAND

Illustrations: KIM DEITCH

HOUGHTON MIFFLIN COMPANY
BOSTON • 1986

Library of Congress Cataloging-in-Publication Data
Lester, Michael.
How to have fun with your body.
1. Group games.   2. Entertaining.   I. Subtle,
Susan.   II. Title.
GV1472.L47   1986   793   86-7622
ISBN 0-395-37934-2

Printed in the United States of America

P 10 9 8 7 6 5 4 3 2 1

Photo credits: Bettmann Archive, 43, 59, 81, 103;
UPI/Bettmann, 12–13; Bettmann Film Archive, 33;
Columbia Pictures, 27; Ed Buryn/Jeroboam, Inc., 92–93;
National Photo and News Service (© E. O. Goldbeck,
San Antonio, Texas), 123.

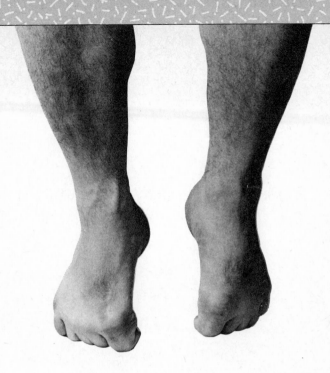

This book is for Don Peterson.
Where other men might knuckle under,
he'd take a stand.

CONTENTS

HOW TO HAVE FUN WITH SOMEONE ELSE'S BODY

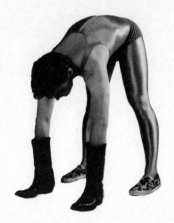

HOW TO HAVE FUN WITH THIS BOOK

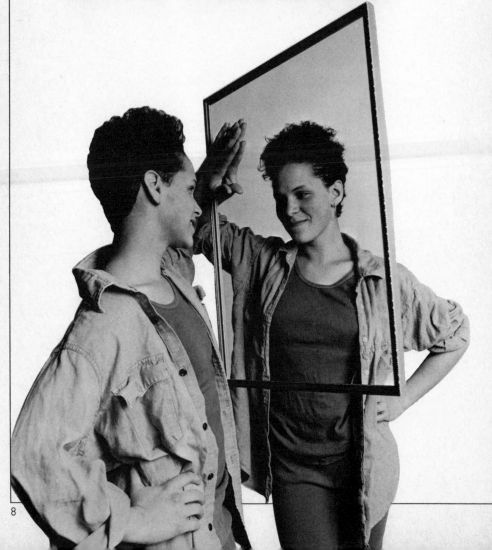

Two rules. Two maxims to live,
love, and learn by. Two for the read.

"One's eyes are what one is."
— John Galsworthy

Rule 1: *Use a mirror.*
Your mirror is your best friend.

If you can't see what you're doing,
how will you know that you're
doing it right?

"I can't take your body
if your heart's not in it."
— Janie Fricke

Rule 2: *Practice.*
Then practice some more.

It's amazing what fun you can have
with your body if only you take
the time to try. Be
patient, be persistent, and please don't get
discouraged. It'll come.
With careful practice, it'll come.

WARNING!!!

Parts of this book may be hazardous to your health.
Please note the DANGER stamp signifying those particularly perilous
exercises where inattention or reckless abandon can lead
to disaster. This woman is a fine example of someone
who wasn't looking where she was going.
And look what happened to her.

Hey, let's be careful out there.

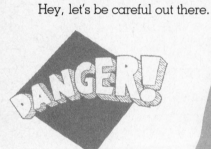

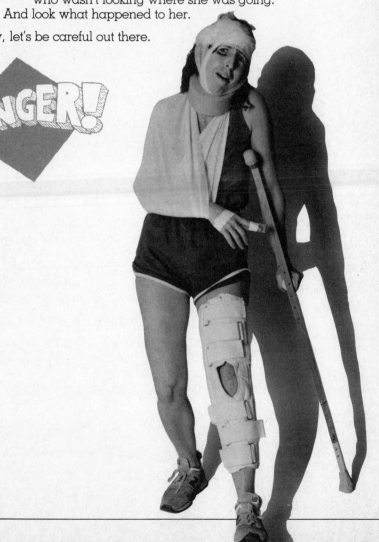

FROM HEAD TO TOE

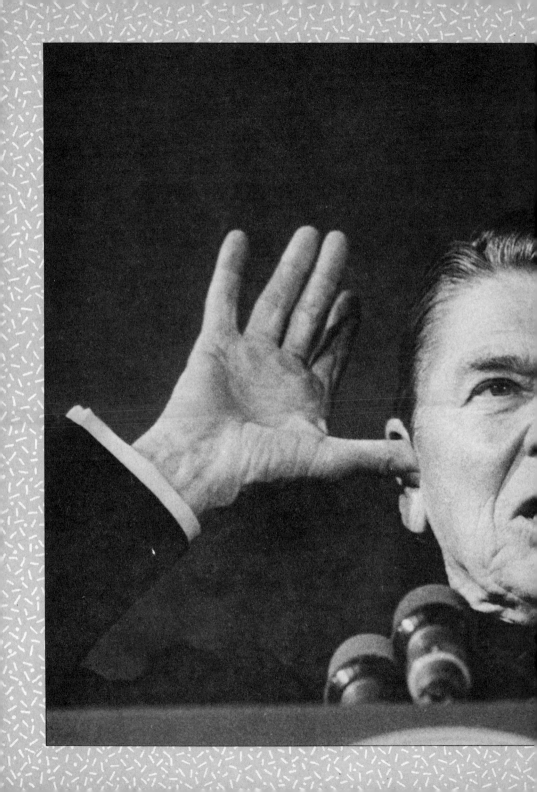

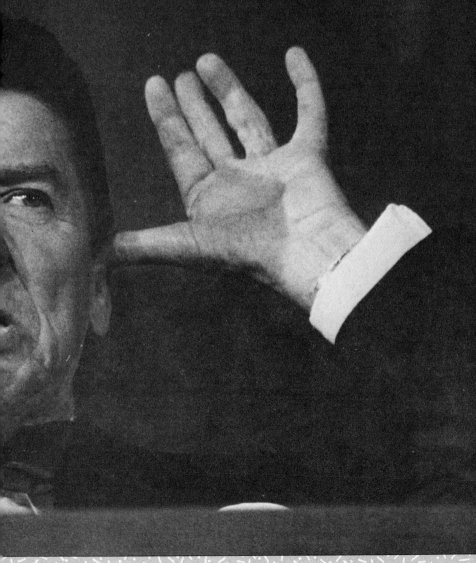

1 WHOLE HEAD

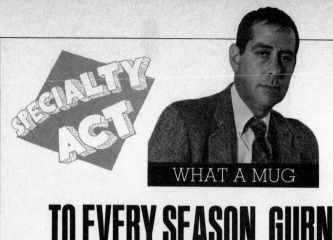

WHAT A MUG

TO EVERY SEASON, GURN, GURN, GURN

A special sort of mugging is known around the Western world as "gurning." Just for the fun of it, fine-looking people turn their faces into the human equivalent of fruits and vegetables.

Every year in Wales there's a gurning competition. Anyone can win, but the English, notorious for their bad teeth and severe underbites, have a distinct advantage. False teeth, you see, provide the face-lift.

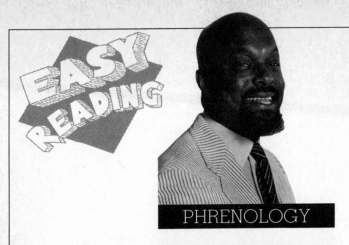

PHRENOLOGY

READ MY MIND

Around 1800, a young German doctor named Franz Joseph Gall had the gall to insist that, by studying the shape of a man's head, he could diagnose the inner man — his emotions, thoughts, and personality. During the nineteenth century, Gall's "science" of phrenology became widely popular. No less a luminary than abolitionist Henry Ward Beecher lectured about its merits and went around the country giving phrenological readings at two cents a head.

In phrenology, the human head is divided into forty-two departments — eleven in a row through the center and thirty-one in pairs on either side — each representing a different trait. If there's a bump or bulge in a particular department, then the individual is skilled in that area. For example, Albert Einstein's head was unusually wide at the outside of the eyes — the area of mathematics; Will Rogers's head had protrusions above the outer edge of his eyebrows — the area of mirthfulness; explorer Roald Amundsen's forehead bulged in the middle — the area of locality, or sense of direction.

Scientists today consider this kind of evaluation to be misdirected and superficial. A comparison of a phrenologist's map of the brain with the actual findings of neurologists shows no correspondence either in the location or in the function of brain areas represented. But what do scientists know? Equipped with a phrenological chart (see next two pages), you can feel and thus see for yourself just who is ahead in this Battle of the Bulge.

Departments of the Brain:
1. Observation
2. Eventuality (memory of events)
3. Comparison (discrimination)
4. Causality (originality)
5. Mirthfulness
6. Locality (sense of direction)
7. Timing
8. Music
9. Mathematics
10. Organization
11. Color
12. Weight
13. Size
14. Form (remembrance of faces)
15. Language
16. Humanity

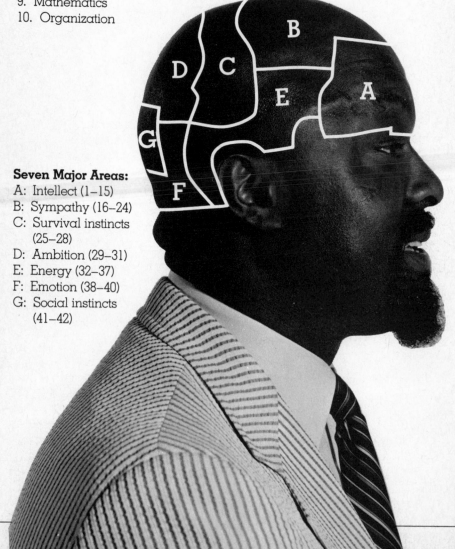

Seven Major Areas:
A: Intellect (1–15)
B: Sympathy (16–24)
C: Survival instincts (25–28)
D: Ambition (29–31)
E: Energy (32–37)
F: Emotion (38–40)
G: Social instincts (41–42)

17. Benevolence
18. Veneration
19. Agreeableness
20. Imitativeness
21. Spirituality
22. Hope
23. Ideality

24. Sublimity
25. Firmness
26. Conscientiousness
27. Caution
28. Secretiveness
29. Self-esteem
30. Approbativeness
31. Continuity
32. Constructive energy
33. Acquisitiveness
34. Appetite
35. Attention to details
36. Aggressiveness
37. Vitality (love of life)
38. Friendship
39. Matrimony
40. Romance
41. Love of home
42. Parental love

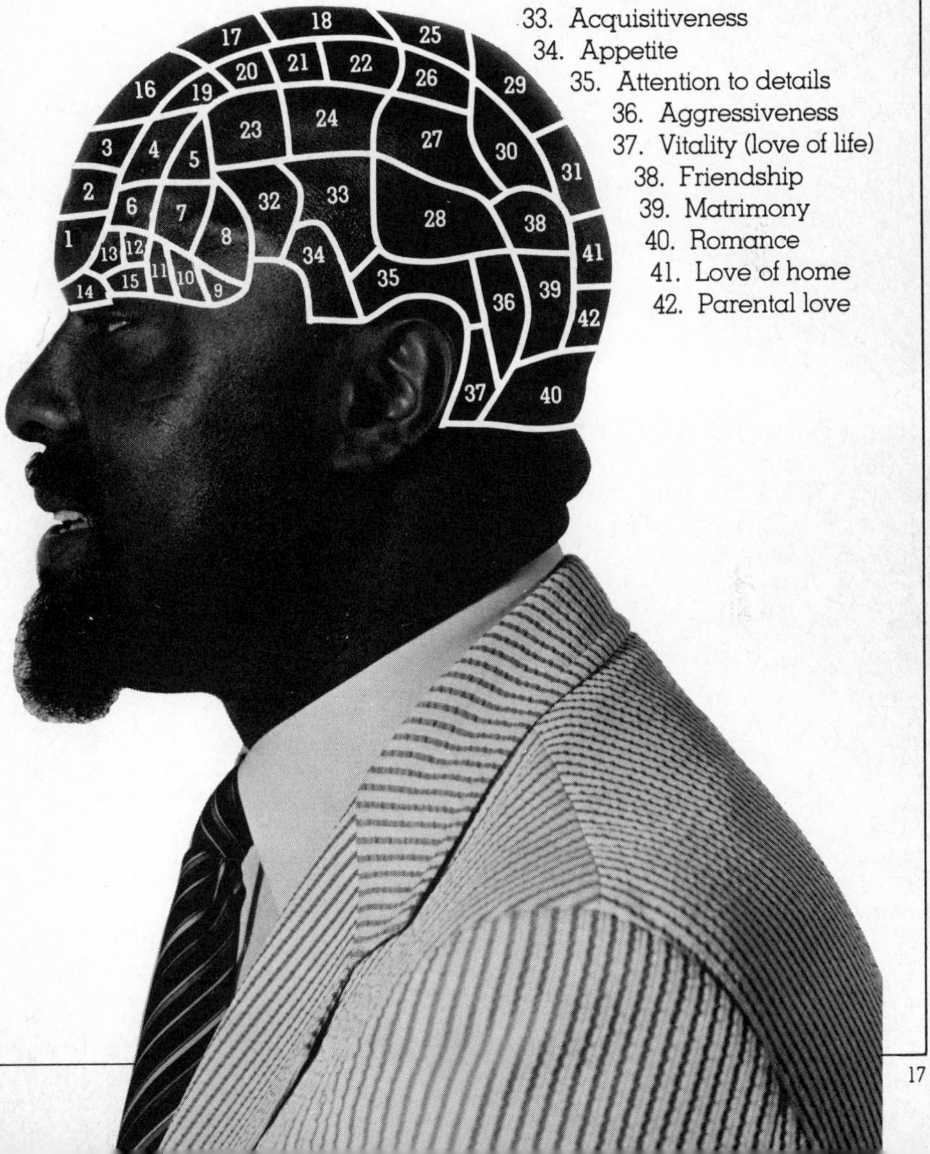

HOW TO BRING OUT THE ANIMAL IN YOU

When the wool is pulled over your eyes, do you feel like a subject on *Wild Kingdom*? Do loved ones call you Lambchops but you're too sheepish to give a *baaa*?

Hey! Let loose those animal instincts.
Put on a funny face. The world is waiting for ewe.

WILD BORE

Wiggle your tongue and use your thumbs to widen your eyes. Snort.

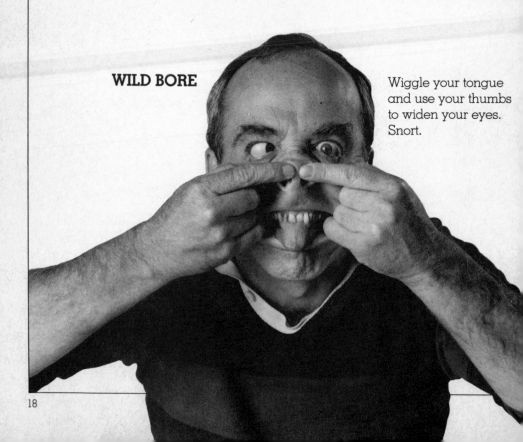

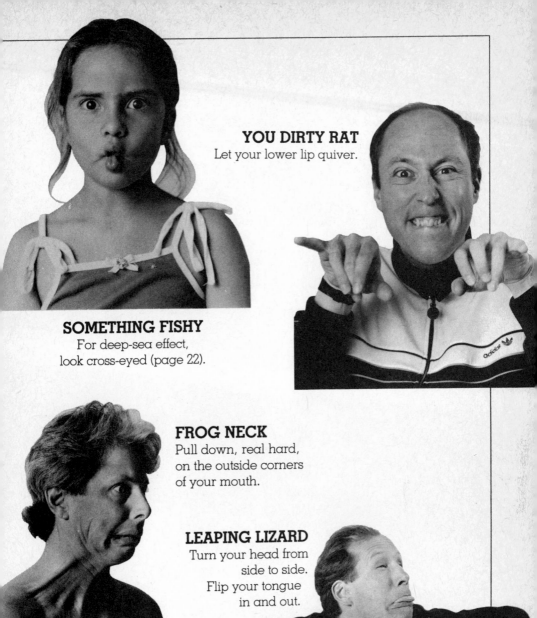

YOU DIRTY RAT
Let your lower lip quiver.

SOMETHING FISHY
For deep-sea effect,
look cross-eyed (page 22).

FROG NECK
Pull down, real hard,
on the outside corners
of your mouth.

LEAPING LIZARD
Turn your head from
side to side.
Flip your tongue
in and out.

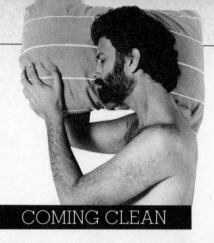

HAIR TODAY, GONE TOMORROW

While sleeping, the average person loses
dozens — sometimes hundreds — of hairs from all over his body.
Here's a nightmare: What would happen if the hairs
came from the same place?

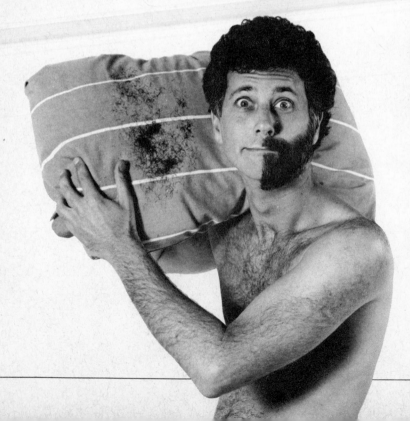

2 EYES

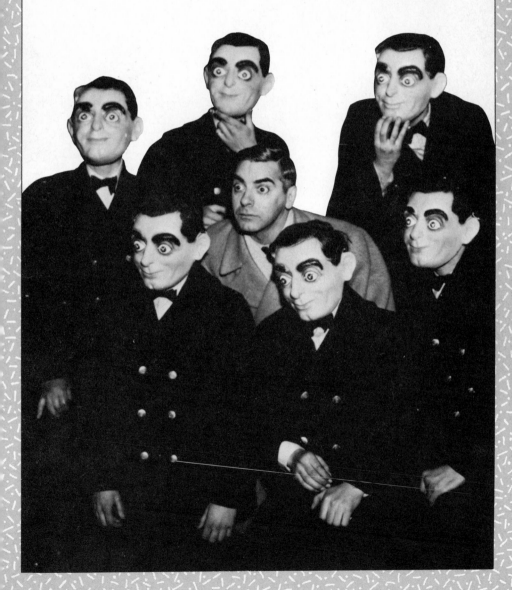

LET'S SEE IF WE CAN MEET MIDWAY ON THIS

Hold your index finger at arm's length. Point it at the bridge of your nose. With both eyes focused on it, slowly **move** your **finger toward your face.** Maintain a single image of your finger. Don't let it go double on you. At a certain point (about 4 inches away) your eyes will cross. They *will* cross.

At this point, you'll feel your eyes straining and a terrible headache coming on. Great! Hold your finger there; cultivate that sensation. Eventually you'll be able to cross your eyes without resorting to such finger-pointing tactics.

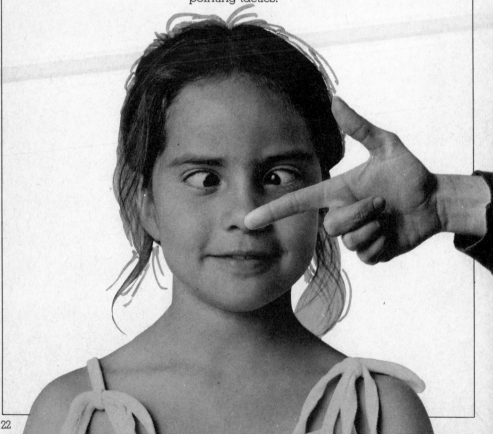

HOW TO FLIP YOUR LID

Somewhere, deep down where you live, your sub-subconscious will be revulsed and repulsed when you try to turn your eyelid inside out. Relax. Don't fight it. Tell yourself that it won't hurt a bit (it won't, really). Try a little reverse psychology.

First, firmly grasp your eyelash and, looking downward, pull your eyelid away from your eyeball. Then, pull the eyelash up and use your eye muscles to close your eye. Immediately let go of your lash.

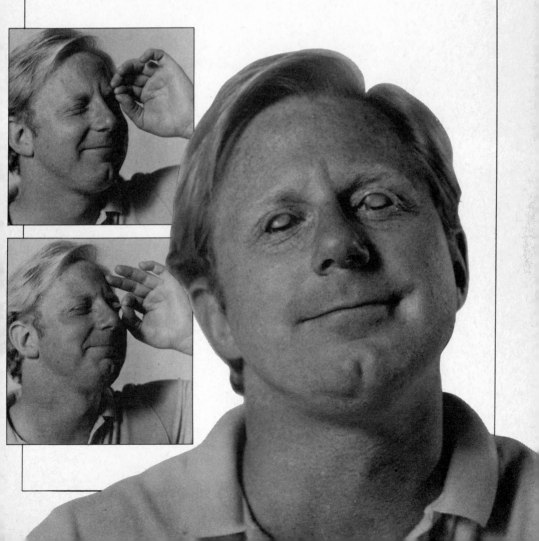

HOW TO GIVE THE EYE, PART I

As flirtation rituals go, giving the eye is a given. Personal idiosyncrasies abound, but this lingering eye movement is the first step in most mating games. You can pick up a stranger across a crowded room or while sharing a seat on the bus . . . You can condense a mountain of monologue into a mere moment.

Here's how The Look looks:

THE GUY:

Your eyebrows rise quizzically, your smile softly broadens. Pervading your entire expression is that silly smirk of awkward expectation.

THE GAL:

Not simultaneously (maybe before, probably after), you peek and peer through your eyelashes — out the sides or shyly downward. You're sultry, of course, but there's a certain coyness, perhaps a slight pout about the mouth, just in case you get rejected.

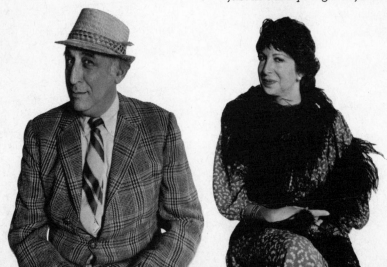

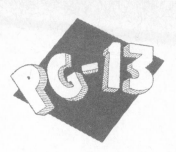

PG-13

"Keep your eye clear and hit 'em where they ain't."
— William ("Wee Willie") Keeler

Direct Eye Contact
The given eye has been gotten. Show the euphoria you're feeling. Smile. Then quickly say something nice.

Too much work? Turn the page and . . .

BINGO!

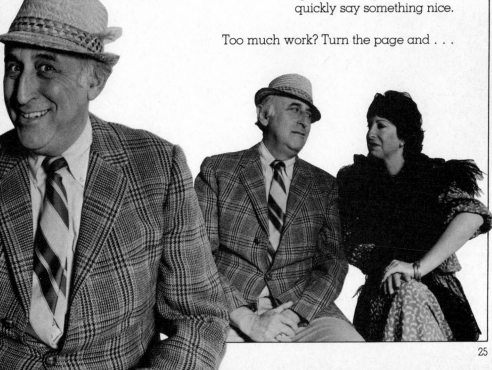

HOW TO GIVE THE EYE, PART II

There are times in your life when you need a quick pick-me-up, when you feel flirtatious.

You **wink,** therefore you are.

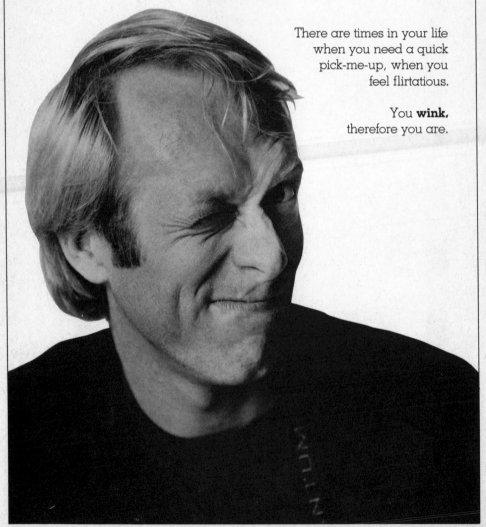

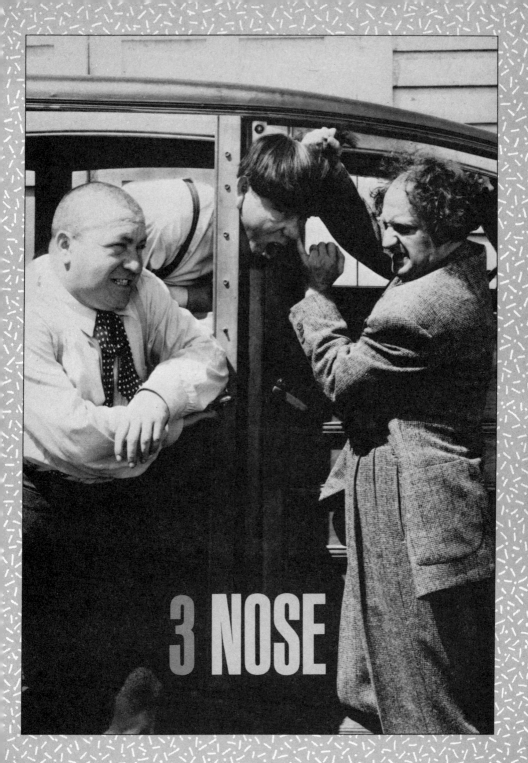

3 NOSE

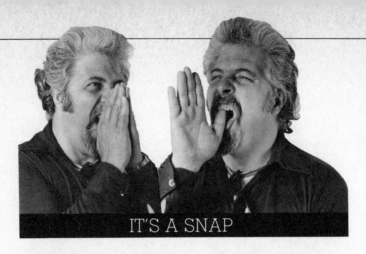

HOW TO BREAK YOUR NOSE

Actually, it's: How to Fool Innocent People into Thinking That You're Breaking Your Nose.

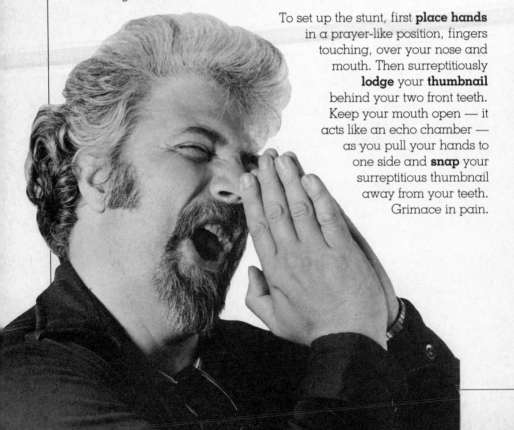

To set up the stunt, first **place hands** in a prayer-like position, fingers touching, over your nose and mouth. Then surreptitiously **lodge** your **thumbnail** behind your two front teeth. Keep your mouth open — it acts like an echo chamber — as you pull your hands to one side and **snap** your surreptitious thumbnail away from your teeth. Grimace in pain.

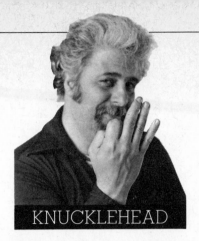

KNUCKLEHEAD

HOW TO PICK YOUR NOSE

"When you get there, send me a postcard."
— Anonymous

First, bend your index
finger at the second joint.
Then, stick the joint
in your nostril.

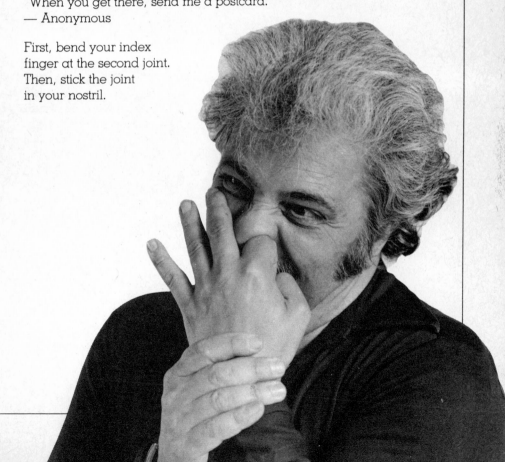

BALANCING ACT

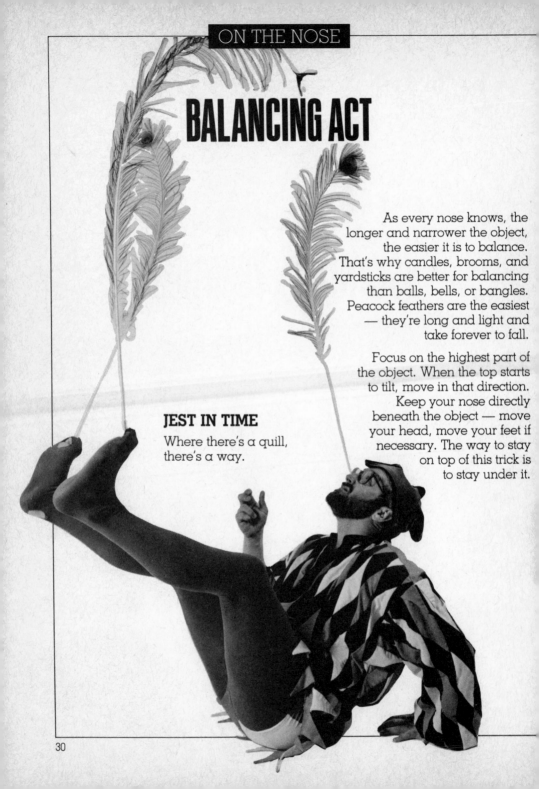

As every nose knows, the longer and narrower the object, the easier it is to balance. That's why candles, brooms, and yardsticks are better for balancing than balls, bells, or bangles. Peacock feathers are the easiest — they're long and light and take forever to fall.

Focus on the highest part of the object. When the top starts to tilt, move in that direction. Keep your nose directly beneath the object — move your head, move your feet if necessary. The way to stay on top of this trick is to stay under it.

JEST IN TIME

Where there's a quill, there's a way.

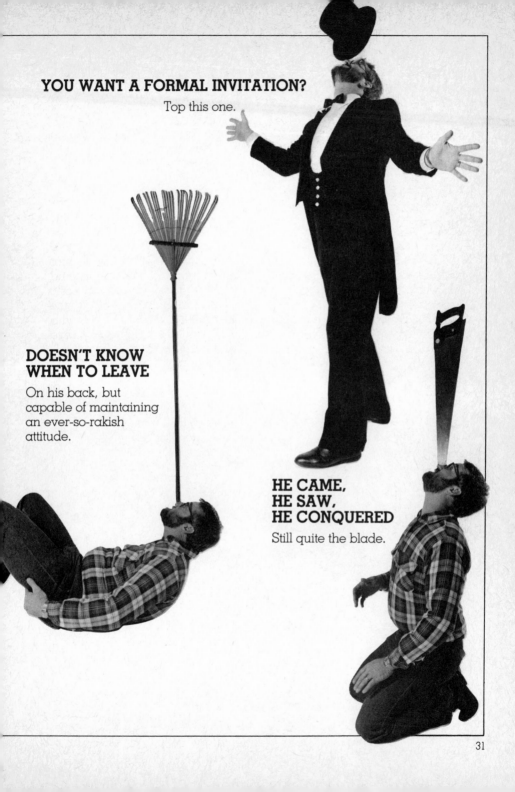

YOU WANT A FORMAL INVITATION?

Top this one.

DOESN'T KNOW WHEN TO LEAVE

On his back, but capable of maintaining an ever-so-rakish attitude.

HE CAME, HE SAW, HE CONQUERED

Still quite the blade.

POP QUIZ

TRUE OR FALSE: In phrenology, the sign of a great lover is a big bump at the back of the head, just above the collar.

True. It's "the bulge of romance."

MULTIPLE CHOICE:
When you demonstrate to your closest friends what you've learned so far, they
A. Call the cops.
B. Knit brows and roll eyes.
C. Take it on the chin.
D. Wink right back.
E. All of the above, all at the same time.

D. Right back, and then left back.

DISCUSSION QUESTIONS:
A. Why do you have ear lobes?
B. If the whites of your eyes weren't white, what color would they be?
C. Take off your clothes and study yourself in the mirror. Forget it. Put your clothes back on.

IDENTIFICATION:
This man is sporting a
A. Fu mushu fork.
B. French kiss.
C. Beer-foam strainer.
D. Double-longhorn mustache.

(For French kiss, see page 83.)
D. Made in Texas.

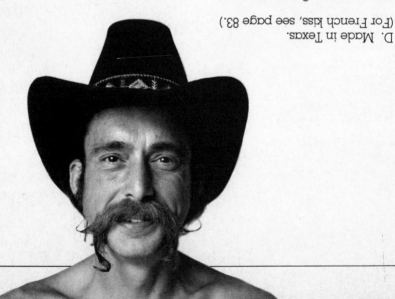

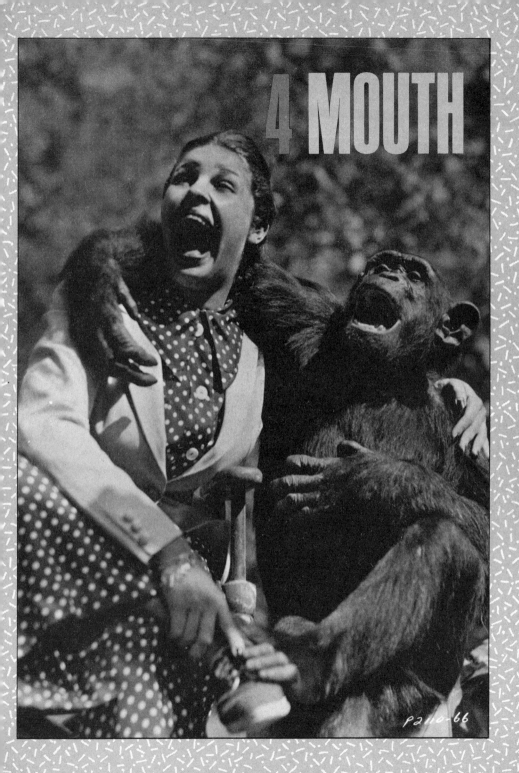

4 MOUTH

P2110-66

LIVING HAND TO MOUTH

Some people bite off more than they can chew. So don't try this trick unless you have a small hand and a big mouth. Wedge your fingers first, then squeeze in your thumb. Understand?

Rrrgruggurruh.

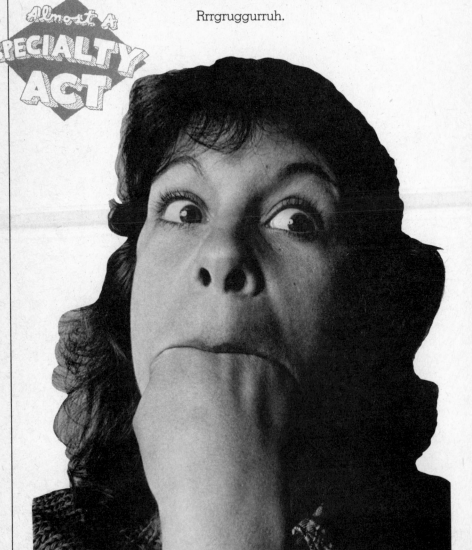

Almost A **SPECIALTY ACT**

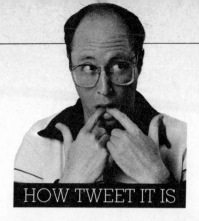

THE TWO-FINGER WHISTLE

Place the tips of your index fingers together at a 90-degree angle. Press them against the tip of your tongue, rolling it upward and backward. Close your lips over the first joints. Make certain that your lips are drawn tightly over your teeth.

Move the tips of your fingers a silly centimeter apart. **Blow** briskly and steadily through this gap.

Experiment until you get it right. Move your fingers closer together or farther apart; vary the angle. Many whistlers prefer to use their thumb and index finger. Some even use four fingers, but that's a real mouthful for beginners.

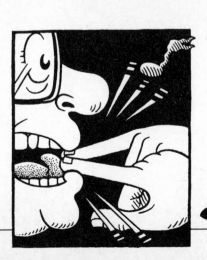

ORAL EXAM

You are born with the tongue your parents gave you.
Which of these tongue tricks is inherited?

1. Curl   5. Double Cloverleaf
2. Chin Lick   6. Left Turn
3. Right Turn   7. Nose Pick
4. Cloverleaf   8. All of the above

1.

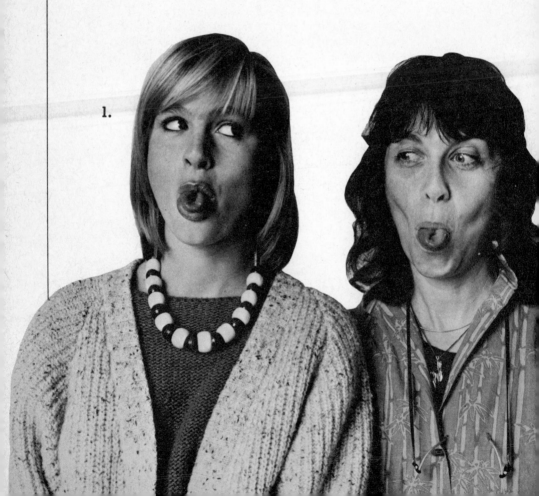

ANSWER: 9. None of the above. (This is a trick question.)
Genetic researchers think that some twists of the tongue are
inherited, but they're wrong.

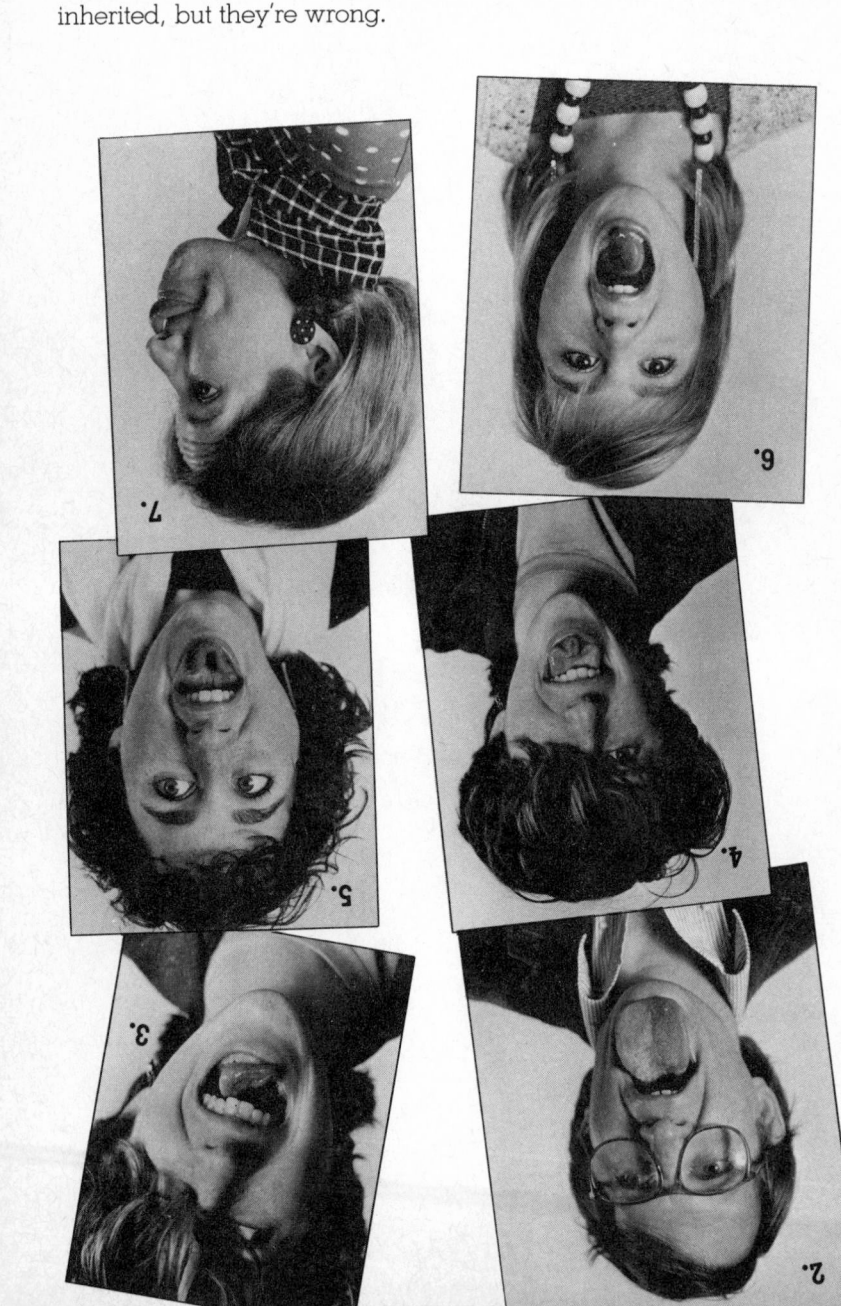

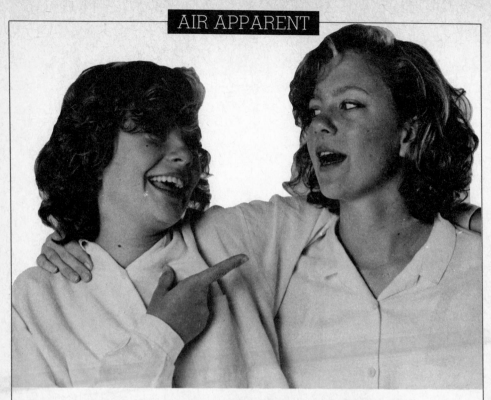

FOREVER BLOWING BUBBLES

Collect about ¼ teaspoon of saliva in the trough behind your bottom front teeth. Pull your tongue back slowly until a tiny globule forms between the tip of your tongue and the back of your lower teeth. Cup your tongue slightly, **scoop** up the bubble, and gently **sigh.** It should slide to the tip of your tongue and, like all good bubbles, burst. But you can always blow another.

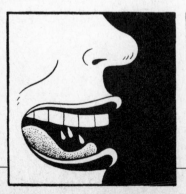 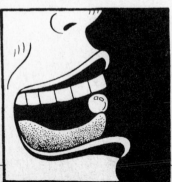

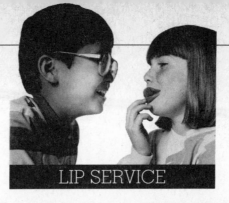

MAKE A MONKEY OF YOURSELF

Kids call this "Monkey Lips." Monkey see? Good. Now, monkey do:

Pout. Pucker up and frown as hard as you can. Curl your lower lip out and down, pulling your chin back with your neck and jaw muscles. (When you practice, it may help to "cheat" by holding your lip down with a finger.) Now, simply **curl** your tongue over your upper lip.

Hint: Tension is the key, so don't laugh. The moment you relax, it all falls apart.

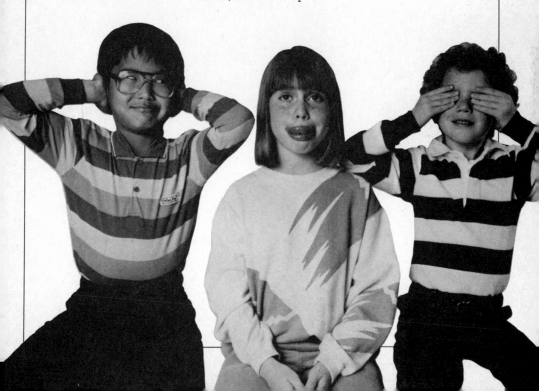

LOOSE LIPS
SEEM SLIPPED

Eat a box of dry cereal, a handful of pretzels, and a dozen salted crackers. When your mouth feels as dry as a dust bowl, pull your lips in opposite directions. Sit perfectly still and look stupid.

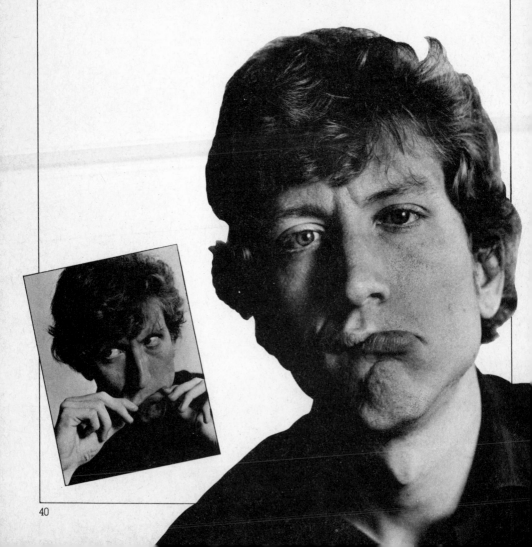

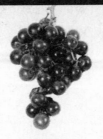

HOW TO THROW A PARTY

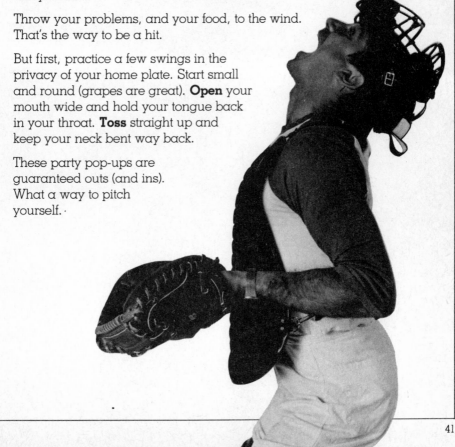

You're at a party where everyone seems to be batting a thousand. But you stand alone—munching on nuts, raisins, cheese cubes—stuck in right field. It's time to impress the other guests. What will you do? What will you do?

Throw your problems, and your food, to the wind. That's the way to be a hit.

But first, practice a few swings in the privacy of your home plate. Start small and round (grapes are great). **Open** your mouth wide and hold your tongue back in your throat. **Toss** straight up and keep your neck bent way back.

These party pop-ups are guaranteed outs (and ins). What a way to pitch yourself. ·

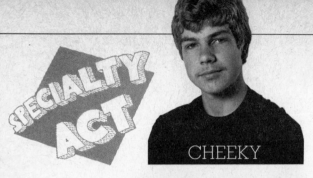

CHEEKY

YOUNG FELLOW WITH A LOT OF PULL

It takes a stretch
of the imagination.

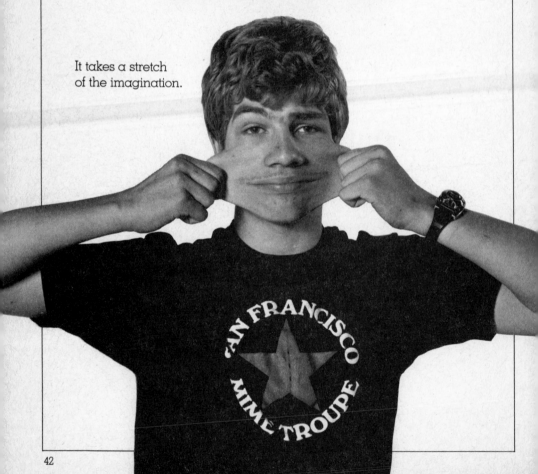

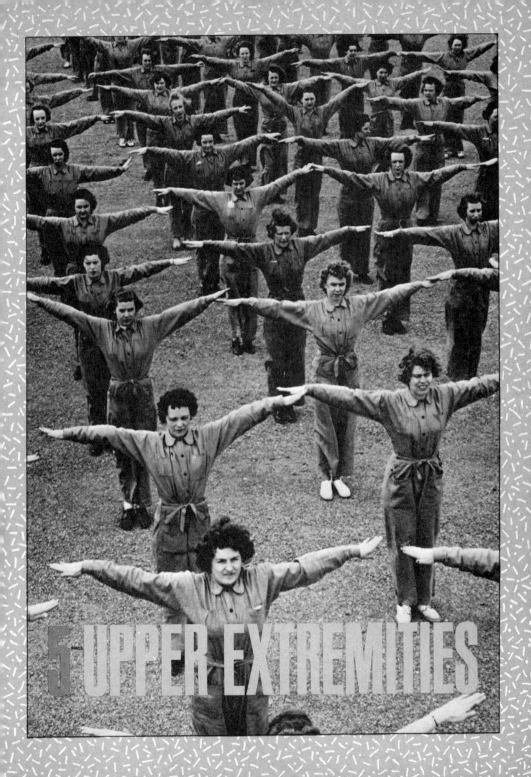

5 UPPER EXTREMITIES

A PIZZA DI ACTION

There are more than 150 manual "words" in the traditional gestural vocabulary of a southern Italian. As they say, tie an Italian's hands behind his back . . . and he's speechless.

"I INSULT YOUR MANHOOD!"
Corna: the sign of a cuckold; the horns of a castrated bull. Jab the index and little fingers accusingly in the air.

"UP YOURS!" Forearm Jerk:
rejection, hostility, the threat of violence. Bend your arm, grab your bicep, and thrust your fist in the air.

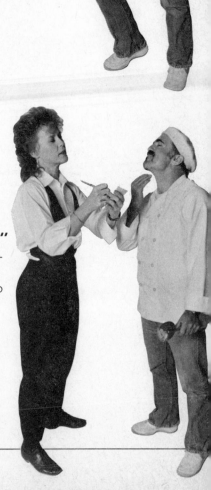

"BUG OFF!"
Chin Flick: a mild form of rejection. Scrape your throat, from the Adam's apple up to the tip of the chin, with your fingernails.

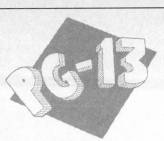

"I CUT YOUR THROAT!"

Throat Cut: aggression. Draw your index finger across your windpipe.

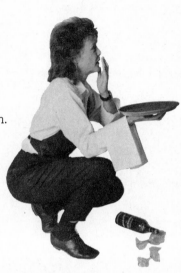

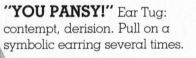

"YOU PANSY!" Ear Tug: contempt, derision. Pull on a symbolic earring several times.

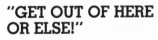

"GET OUT OF HERE OR ELSE!"

Forearm Slap: expulsion. While jerking arm slightly upward, pat it midway between wrist and elbow.

HOW TO GIVE THE FINGER, PART I

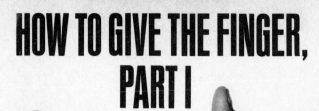

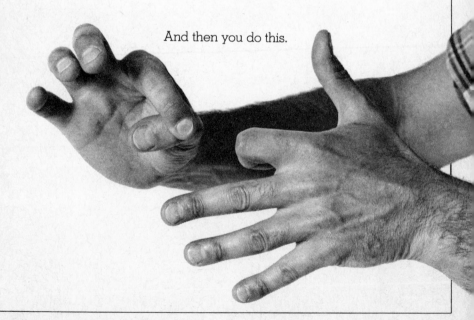

First you do this . . .

And then you do this.

YOU'RE OK, I'M OK, BUT MY HAND HURTS LIKE HELL

The fincle is suited for people with short fingernails. It requires practice, patience, and a willingness to suffer pain. The first few times you try this exercise, your fingertips will probably slide off the ridges and out of place. Make 'em stick.

Place the tip of your little finger (1) on the ridge of your ring finger midway between joints. If it stays there, (2) place the tip of your ring finger between the joints of your middle finger. (3) Place the tip of your middle finger on your index finger as far back as possible. (4) Make a circle with your thumb and index finger. Now that's a fincle, okay?

Okay!

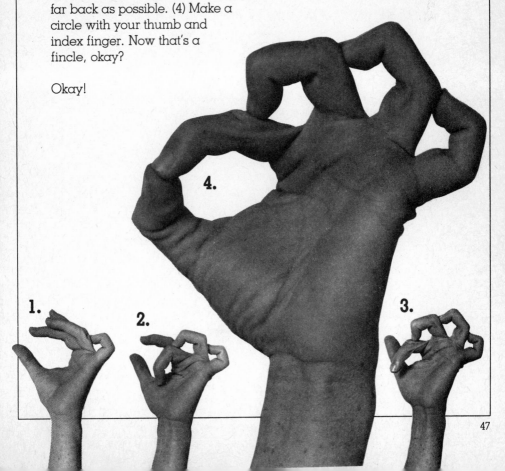

4.

1.

2.

3.

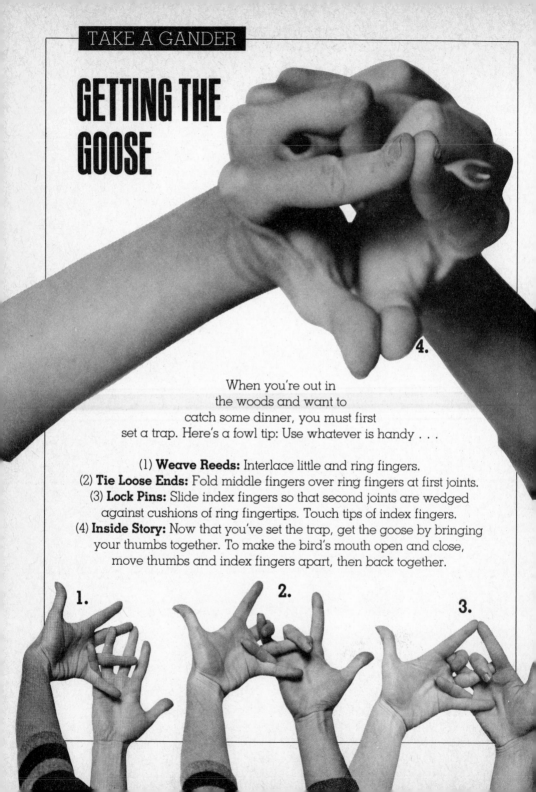

GETTING THE GOOSE

When you're out in
the woods and want to
catch some dinner, you must first
set a trap. Here's a fowl tip: Use whatever is handy . . .

(1) **Weave Reeds:** Interlace little and ring fingers.
(2) **Tie Loose Ends:** Fold middle fingers over ring fingers at first joints.
(3) **Lock Pins:** Slide index fingers so that second joints are wedged
against cushions of ring fingertips. Touch tips of index fingers.
(4) **Inside Story:** Now that you've set the trap, get the goose by bringing
your thumbs together. To make the bird's mouth open and close,
move thumbs and index fingers apart, then back together.

HOW TO RISE TO THE OCCASION

Don't be shy, folks. Grab this chance to watch your very arm float upward against your will! Yes, you too can stare in amazement as your hand hovers mysteriously in space!

Press your whole **arm** against a wall (or lie on it sideways on the floor) for ten minutes or more. You'll start to grimace in discomfort as blood flows out of your increasingly limp limb. Then step away from the wall (or get up off the floor), relax, close your eyes, and **feel** your **arm rise** up, up, and away.

Oh, sure, you're asking, "Is it worth the price of admission, the ten minutes of torture?" Hey, this is a cheap thrill. See for yourself! You have nothing to lose but your self-control.

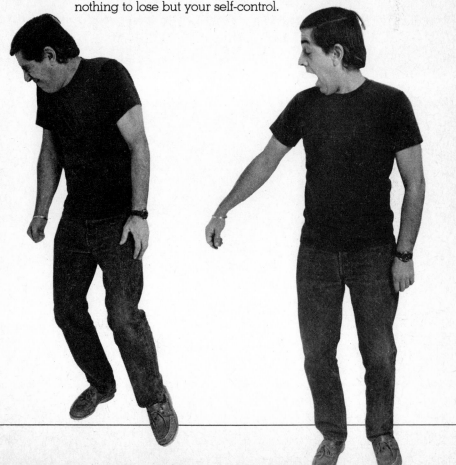

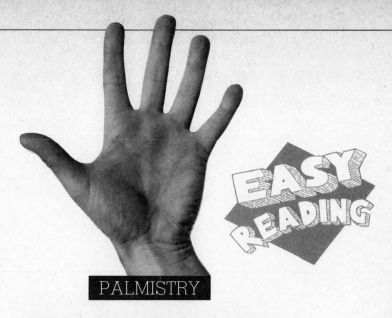

PALMISTRY

WHAT'S YOUR LINE?

Like fingerprints, all palms are unique.
Even your right palm is different from your left palm.
Supposedly, the left hand reveals the characteristics you are
born with, and the right how you put these traits to use.
(For left-handers, this rule is reversed.)

THUMB

Large phalange of Will:
   Person of action.
Large phalange of Reason:
   Philosopher.
Thumbs that can be bent back
toward forearm: Easygoing.
Stiff thumbs:
   Set in one's ways.

FINGERS

Large gaps between fingers:
   Extravagant, unable to save.
Long fingers (almost as long
as palm itself): Gregarious.
Very long fingers:
   Idealistic.
Short fingers:
   Lusty sex drive.

MOUNTS

Mounts are raised "mounds" on the palm. They are most significant when they are visually and tactually prominent.

Venus: Warm, sympathetic, lusty.
Jupiter: Ambitious, arrogant.
Saturn: Well-balanced.
Sun: Happy, successful.
Mercury: Good business sense.

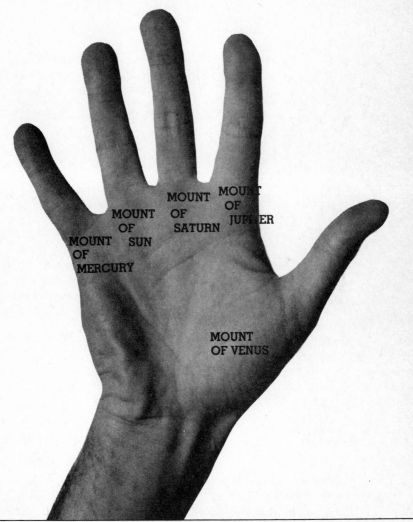

MAJOR LINES OF THE PALM

The healthiest lines are straight and strong, reflecting emotional stamina and mental clarity. Wiggly lines reflect wishy-washy traits. The clearer the line, the more important the information it carries.

LIFE LINE
Short and complex:
Delicacy, ill health.
Broken: Subject to a
life-threatening event.
Branches pointing toward the
fingers: Fame, acclaim.
Double (or parallel) life lines:
A second chance after
illness or disaster.

HEAD LINE
Straight (or slightly sloped),
strong, and long: Brainy.
Slight incline toward wrist:
Astute business sense.
Sudden tilt toward wrist:
Artistic ability.
Long, with lots of slope:
Idealistic, too imaginative.
Tiny gap between head and life
lines at origins (between thumb
and index finger):
Self-contained self-starter.
Large gap: Selfish.
No gap (joined together):
Overly cautious underachiever.

HEART LINE
Running across palm, then up
to mount of Jupiter:
Kindhearted, a good lover.
Broken: A broken heart —
a traumatic romance or,
yes, a heart attack.
Suddenly dipping downward:
Cold, moody, distant.
Fine lines and
branches near
mount of
Saturn, point-
ing toward wrist:
Failures in love.
Fine lines
pointing upward:
Success in love.
Hairlines and branches at
beginning (edge of palm):
Different affairs.

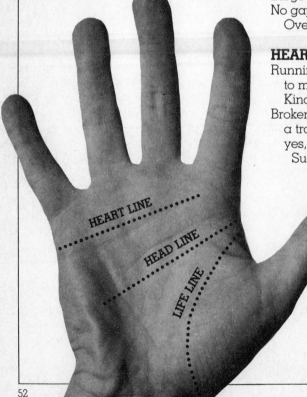

HEART LINE

HEAD LINE

LIFE LINE

MINOR LINES OF THE PALM

LINE OF DESTINY

Long (reaching up to mount of Saturn): Workaholic.

Short (beginning halfway up palm): Unsettled, very directionless.

Stopping at head line: Reluctant to take risks.

Stopping at heart line: Relationship (like marriage) stands in way of other achievements.

Missing entirely from palm: Lack of purpose.

SUN LINE

Long and solid: Riches, wishes come true.

Paralleled by lines running to mount of Mercury: Financial success.

Parallel lines clustered under mount of Sun: Dilettante, too many goals.

Running from beneath mount of Mercury to ring finger: Success through partnership.

MARRIAGE LINE

One line: One marriage.

Two lines: Two marriages.

Near heart line: Early marriage.

Wavy: Rocky romance, uncertainty.

Linking with sun line: Very successful marriage.

AFFECTION LINES

Following curve of thumb and running parallel to life line: Ties with relatives.

Running directly to thumb from life line: Romantic relationships (the more lines, the more relationships).

One clearly etched line: An affair in progress.

LINE OF DESTINY

SUN LINE

MARRIAGE LINE

AFFECTION LINES

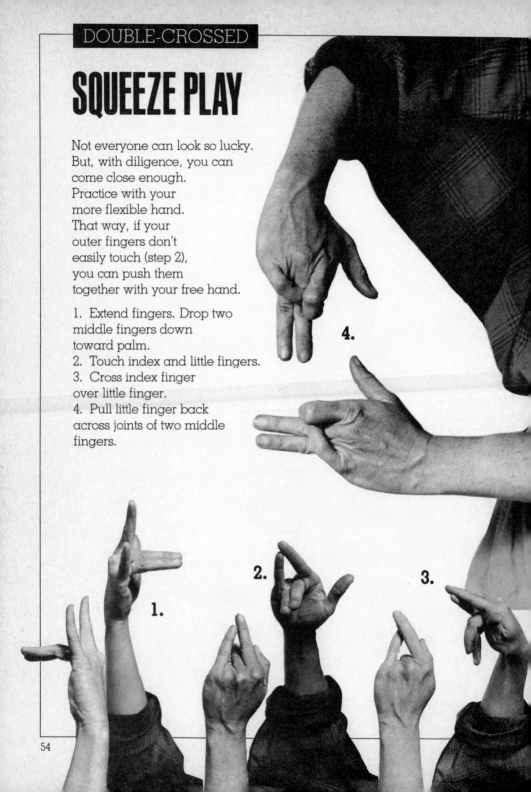

SQUEEZE PLAY

Not everyone can look so lucky. But, with diligence, you can come close enough. Practice with your more flexible hand. That way, if your outer fingers don't easily touch (step 2), you can push them together with your free hand.

1. Extend fingers. Drop two middle fingers down toward palm.
2. Touch index and little fingers.
3. Cross index finger over little finger.
4. Pull little finger back across joints of two middle fingers.

4.

1.

2.

3.

THINGS THAT GO HONK IN THE NIGHT

If the cretinous caveman standing in front of a fire could do it, you can too. You don't need an elaborate stage setup, just a strong light and a white backdrop. The light source should be small but intense; a movie or slide projector is best, but a 100-watt bulb in a cone-shaped lamp works just fine.

Your hands should break into the beam of light about halfway between the light source and the screen. Keep your eyes away from your hands and focus on the screen. Turn off all other lights, pull the curtains, and talk to the animals.

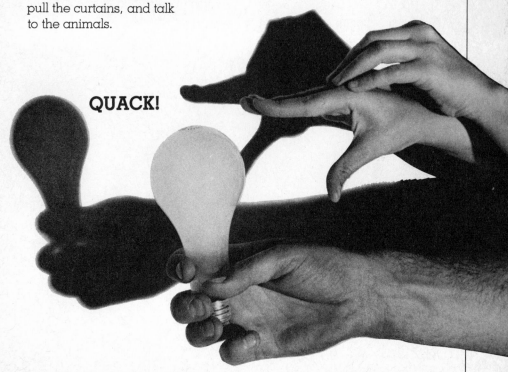

QUACK!

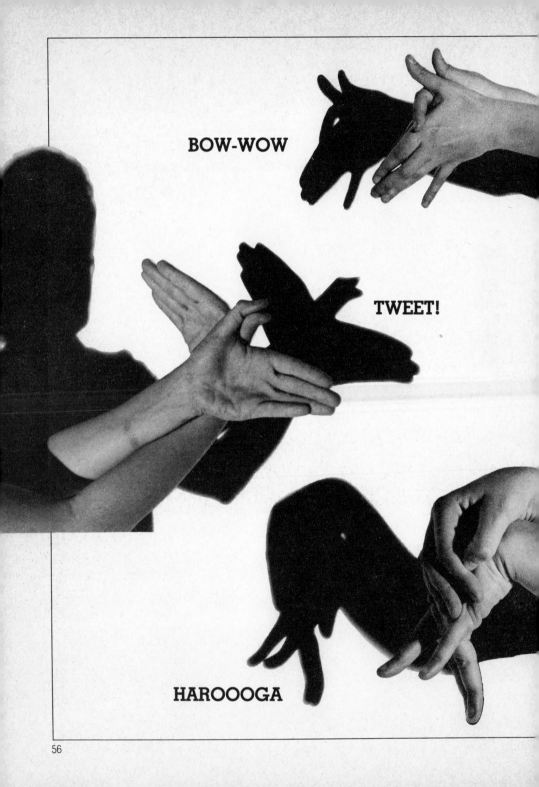

BOW-WOW

TWEET!

HAROOOGA

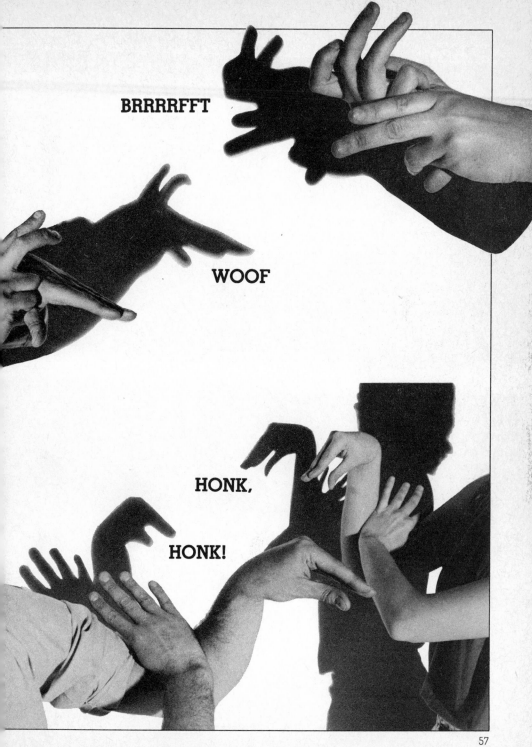

57

HOW TO GIVE THE FINGER, PART II

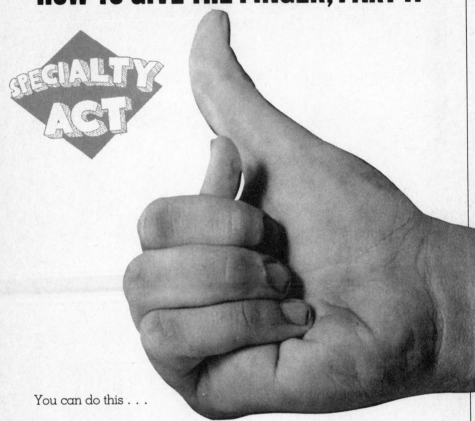

SPECIALTY ACT

You can do this . . .

If you can first do this.

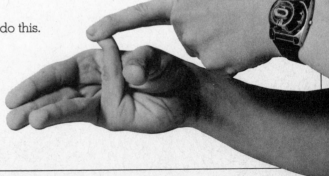

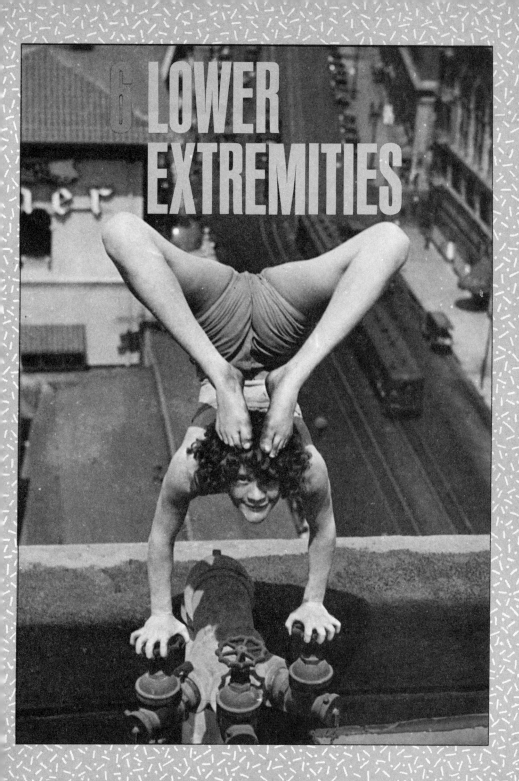

6 LOWER EXTREMITIES

SPLIT PERSONALITY

Week 1:

Stretch those hamstrings. Keep your thighs as close to the ground as possible. If it helps, lean forward.

Practice for fifteen minutes every day for three weeks. Keep it gradual — one step at a time.

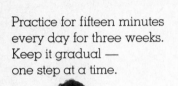

Week 2: Gradually edge your leg forward. For as long as you can handle the pull on your hamstrings (maybe a minute, maybe more), push your body down toward the ground. No pain, no gain.

Week 3:

Voilà! **Spread** the news of your latest feat to your friends. It'll floor them.

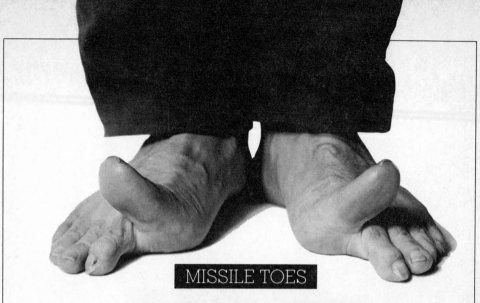

MISSILE TOES

WE'VE GOT LIFTOFF!

Does the idea of splits make you want to split?
Try raising your consciousness.
Start with something small, like your big toes.

As everyone knows, when it comes to toes,

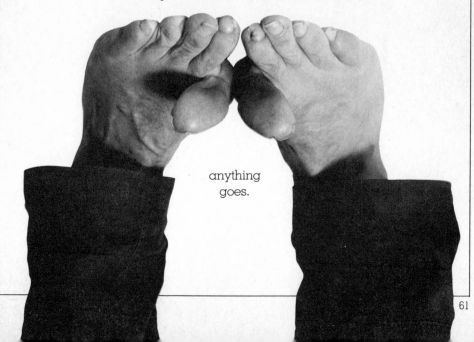

anything
goes.

AYE, HERE'S THE RUB

In 1913, William Fitzgerald of Hartford, Connecticut, introduced reflexology to Western medicine with the claim that internal organs can be stimulated by compressing corresponding areas of the foot. True, foot massage does relieve tension, improve circulation, and relax the entire body. But believing in a direct correlation between areas of the foot and organs of the body, well, that requires some sole searching on your part.

Begin with the toes and work your way down, concentrating on one spot at a time. Use your thumbs and make deep, rolling motions. Vary the amount of pressure from two to ten pounds. (You can practice your pressure performance on a bathroom scale.) Spend extra time on those tender areas, and heel thyself.

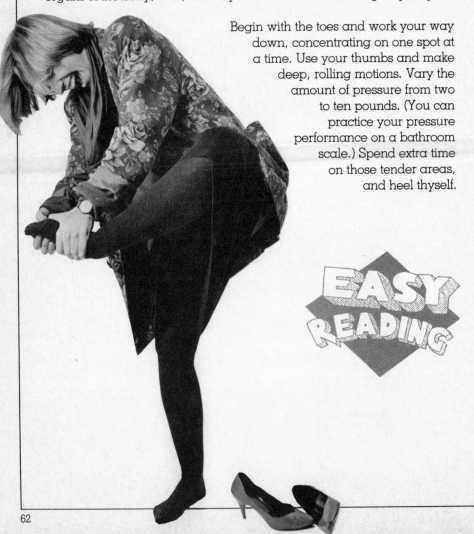

EASY READING

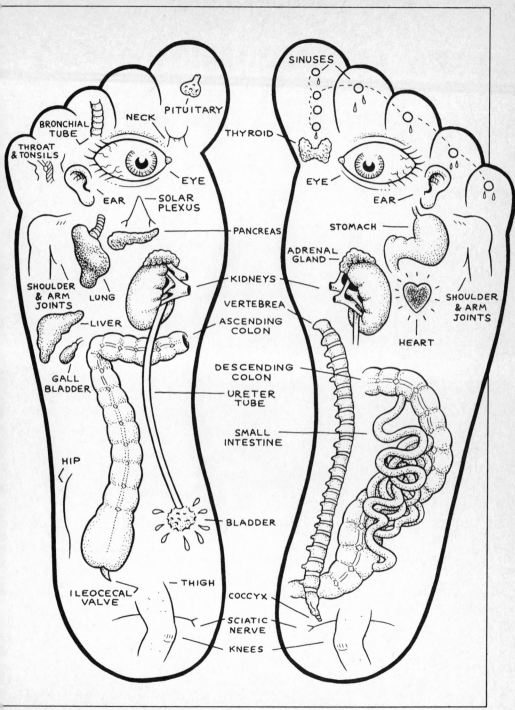

BRONCHIAL TUBE

NECK

PITUITARY

SINUSES

THROAT & TONSILS

THYROID

EAR

EYE

SOLAR PLEXUS

EYE

EAR

PANCREAS

STOMACH

SHOULDER & ARM JOINTS

LUNG

ADRENAL GLAND

KIDNEYS

VERTEBREA

ASCENDING COLON

HEART

SHOULDER & ARM JOINTS

LIVER

GALL BLADDER

DESCENDING COLON

URETER TUBE

SMALL INTESTINE

HIP

BLADDER

ILEOCECAL VALVE

THIGH

COCCYX

SCIATIC NERVE

KNEES

HOW TO PUT YOUR FOOT IN YOUR MOUTH

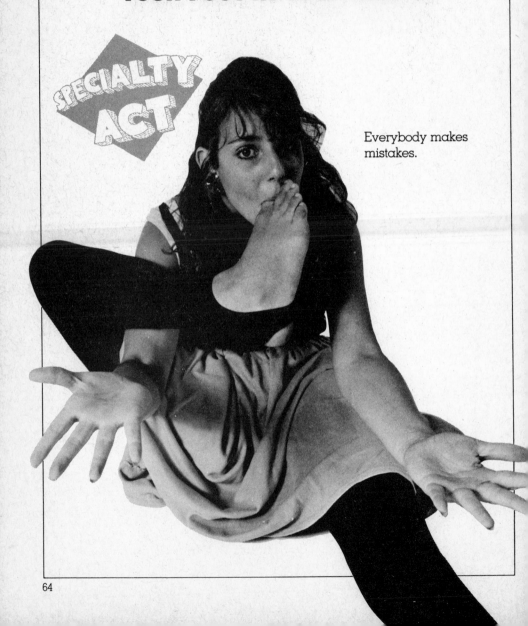

SPECIALTY ACT

Everybody makes mistakes.

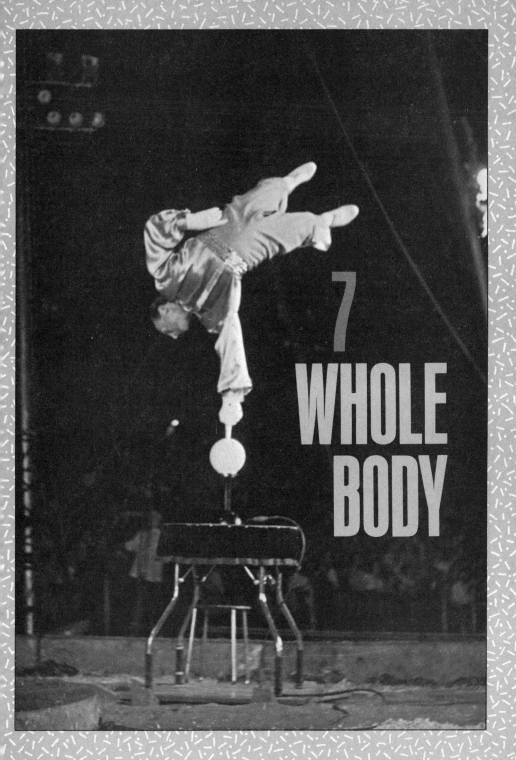

7
WHOLE
BODY

THE MEDIUM IS MASSAGE

Oh, sure, it would be nice to spell relief O-L-G-A (a Swedish masseuse) or K-A-T-S-U (a shiatsu practitioner). But what if there are no Olgas, no Katsus, no acupressurists in your neck of the woods? Apply the pressure yourself. You can be anywhere — on a plane, in a train, at work, watching TV. All you need are some balls.

Tennis balls are best because of their size and resistance, but marbles, golf balls, racquetballs, even baseballs, work wonders. Massage one problem area at a time, and don't overdo it at the first sitting.

To keep everything in balance, work on both sides of your body — if you do the right foot, then do the left foot; if behind the right ear, then behind the left. In no time at all, you'll improve circulation, release stress, and relax muscles. Katsu would be proud of you.

UPPER BACK

Lie on the floor, lean against a wall, or sit against a high-backed chair. Place one or two balls between shoulder blades and spine. Roll balls in problem area for less than a minute.

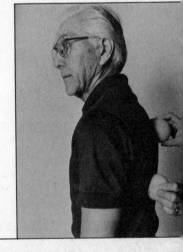

LOWER BACK

Lie on the floor or sit in a chair.
Place one or more balls 1½ to 2 inches
on either side of the spine, anywhere
between the bottom of the shoulder
blades and the waist area. Roll balls
initially for less than a minute.

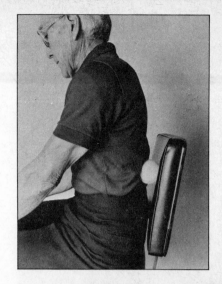

LEGS, LOWER BACK, AND YOU-KNOW-WHAT

Empty your pockets and sit in
a chair. Place one or two balls
in the dimple of your buttocks,
around but not on the bone
you can feel in the middle of each
bun. Roll around on the
balls for 1 to 2 minutes.

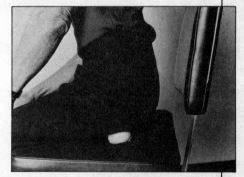

FEET

Sit in a chair. Roll a small
ball or a basket of marbles
under one foot at a time for anywhere from 15 to 30 minutes per foot.

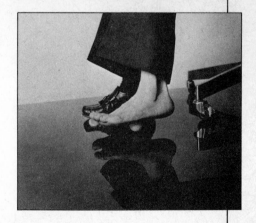

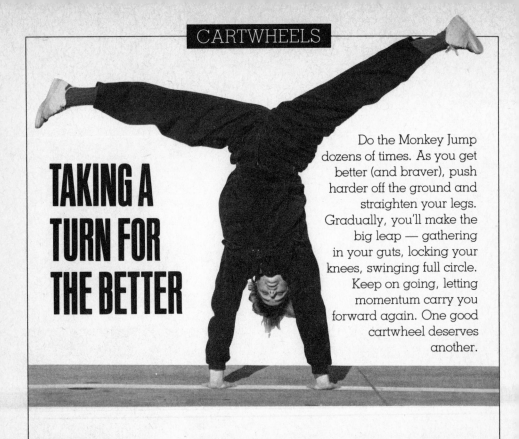

TAKING A TURN FOR THE BETTER

Do the Monkey Jump dozens of times. As you get better (and braver), push harder off the ground and straighten your legs. Gradually, you'll make the big leap — gathering in your guts, locking your knees, swinging full circle. Keep on going, letting momentum carry you forward again. One good cartwheel deserves another.

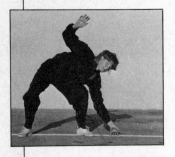
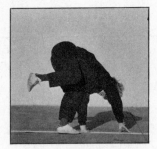
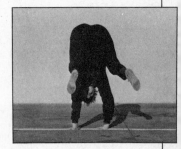

MONKEY JUMP

Squat. Place your dominant hand beside your foot, fingers pointing back. Swing your other hand in an arc over your body and

. . . place it a shoulder's width away. **Kick** your outside leg in a low arc so that it lands on the other side.

As this leg circles, shift your weight. **Jump** around and rise to a standing position, facing in the same direction you started.

IF BELLYBUTTONS COULD TALK

"The way to a man's stomach is through his mouth." — Mrs. Lester

You're relaxing with the family after a big meal, chewing the fat (so to speak), when — without your permission, beyond your control — your stomach starts to growl. What is it saying?

God made the bellybutton as a mouthpiece for the stomach's cares and concerns. So, the next time an embarrassing gurgle escapes your abdomen, expose your umbilical. Let your fingers do the walking and your stomach do the talking. It's a belly laugh.

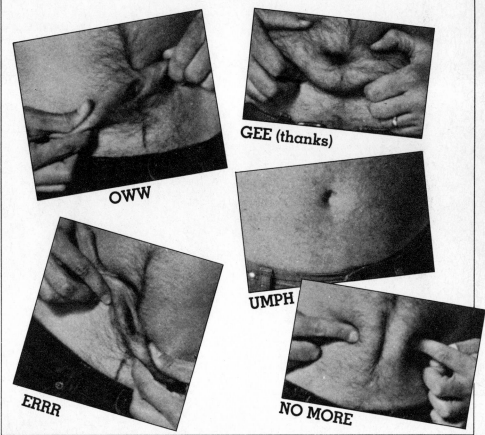

OWW

GEE (thanks)

UMPH

ERRR

NO MORE

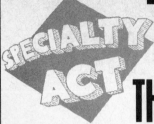

BEAUTY IS IN THE BODY OF THE HOLDER

Great news! A rogue's gallery wants to commission your body paintings. Put yourself in the proper frame of mind and make your life imitate art.

PICASSO

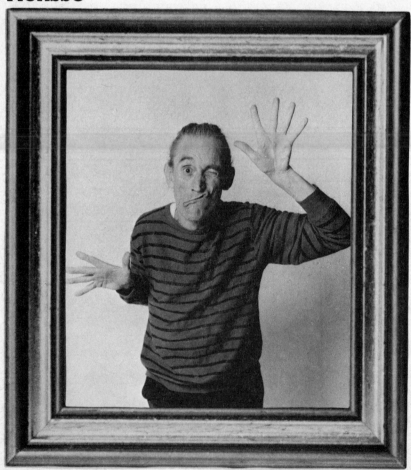

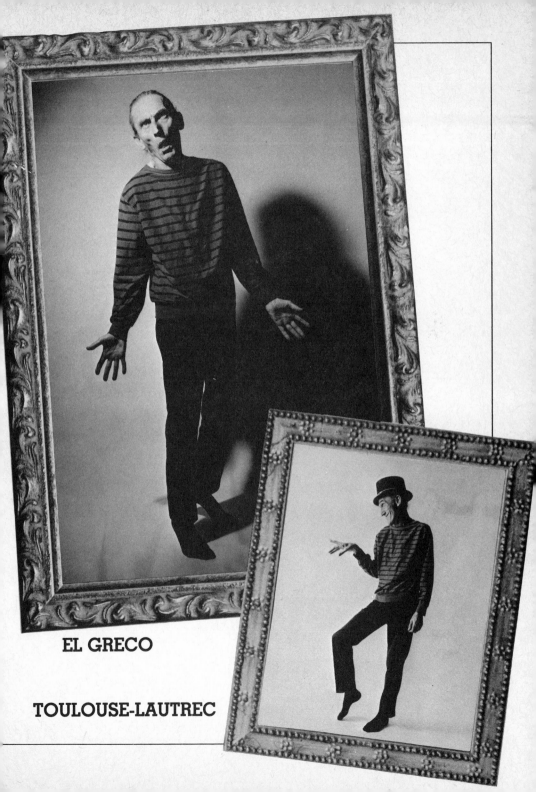

EL GRECO

TOULOUSE-LAUTREC

UP AGAINST THE WALL

Find a nice, big, empty wall. Put a firm pillow 4 to 12 inches from the wall. **Kneel** and rest the top of your head on the pillow.

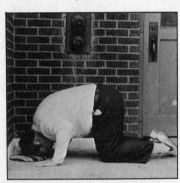

Straighten your legs and come up on your toes.

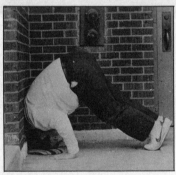

Lift one leg and bring its heel against the wall. **Kick** back the other leg so both heels touch the wall. Straighten your back and legs. **Smile.** Once you get good at this, you might try it without a wall.
Then again, you might not.

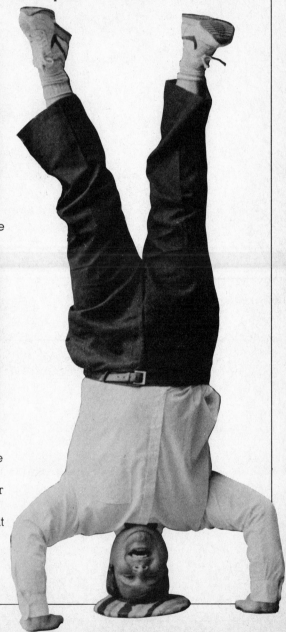

EXCUSE ME, I'M TAKING A POLE...

Hanging horizontally from a pole is a matter of balance, not brute strength. Pick a pole 2 to 3 inches in diameter (the signs at bus stops are perfect). With your stronger arm (say, your right), **grip** the pole at mid-thigh level, palm facing out, fingers pointing down. **Lodge** your right **elbow** in your right pelvic "pocket" — that soft spot just inside your hip.

Your entire weight will end up here, so make it nice and snug. Cross your left hand in front of your chest, swing it counter-clockwise around the pole, and **grip** the pole 6 to 10 inches above your right hand, with the palm away from you. With the pole cradled in your left armpit, **lean** down on your right shoulder. Raise first the left foot, then the right foot, off the ground, easing your weight forward onto your right elbow. If leverage is a problem, alter the distance between your hands.

73

BARELY YOGA

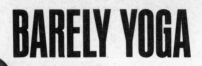

In the age-old art of yoga, there are more than 2,000 prescribed postures aimed at unifying body and mind. These often awkward positions are accompanied by deep meditation, intense concentration, and controlled breathing.

The long-range goal (one that may take several lifetimes) is for the individual to achieve perfect illumination. Through bodily discipline, the individual is eventually liberated from the distractions of the physical world.

The short-range goal is for the individual to keep the diaper from falling off.

THE STORK

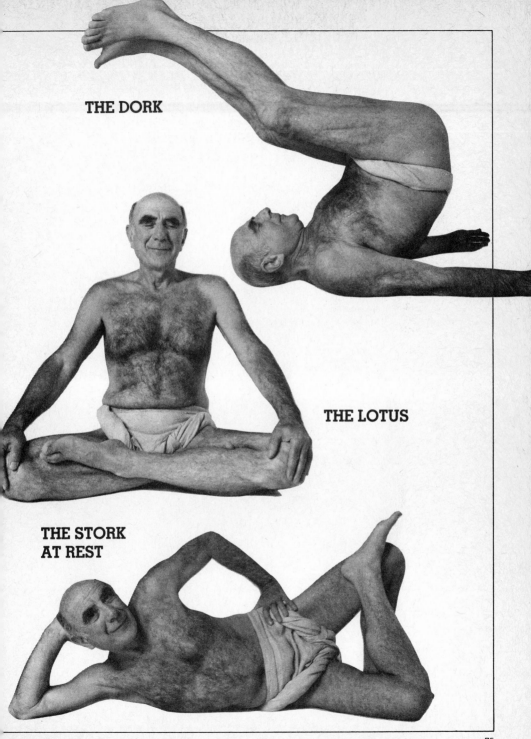

THE DORK

THE LOTUS

THE STORK
AT REST

HOW TO STRETCH OUT YOUR COFFEE BREAK

Take the drain out of workday drudgery. In a matter of minutes, you can loosen up physically and tighten up mentally. Take slow, deep breaths throughout, exhaling whenever you bend. Do each exercise, relax, then, if you have the time, do them all again.

Note: If your office chair has wheels, hold on to your desk or plant your feet firmly. Otherwise, you'll give new meaning to the term "young executive on the go."

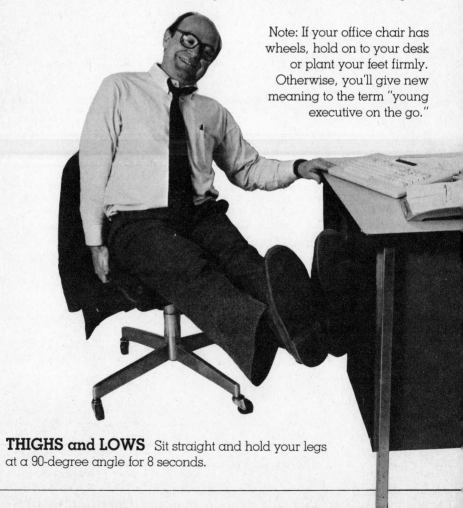

THIGHS and LOWS Sit straight and hold your legs at a 90-degree angle for 8 seconds.

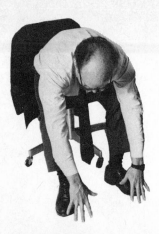

WRISTY BUSINESS
With elbow on desk, pull your wrist back. Hold for 8 seconds, then repeat with other hand.

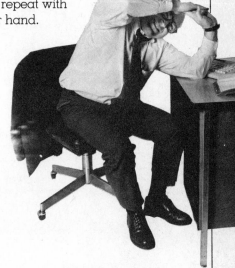

BACKBONE OF THE COMPANY
Bend over between your knees as far as you can go. Hold for a count of 8 seconds, then straighten up slowly. Repeat, reaching farther toward the floor.

SUCCESSFUL MERGER
Bring your right hand down and your left hand up, and try to hook fingers. Hold for 8 seconds, then switch hands and repeat.

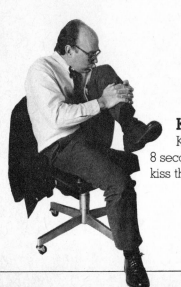

KNEEDY CAUSE
Kiss one knee for 8 seconds, then kiss the other one.

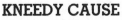
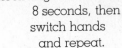

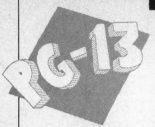

PG-13

INTERNATIONAL DENUNCIATION GUIDE

Every culture has its own insulting gestures. Before traveling to a foreign land, familiarize yourself with the appropriate signs of abuse. Familiarity breeds contempt.

British: "Go have sex with yourself." Reverse the V-for-Victory sign.

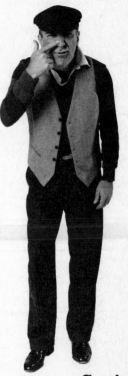

Greek:
"You can say whatever you like, but I'm going to do what I want, so there." Literally, "You can put a hole in my nose."

Arabic:
"What you're saying isn't worth listening to." Literally, "The applause of my thumbnail signifies the value of your company."

Scandinavian:
"One more word out of you and I may have to be impolite." Occasionally followed by a stifled yawn.

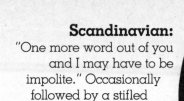

French:
"Que dalle."
Literally, "What a worthless bit of floor tiling."
A forceful flicking of the thumbnail off the upper front teeth.

Bronx:
"You're a bum." Literally, "Pppppppppppffft." A fluttering of the tongue between the lips, a.k.a. "the raspberry."

HOW TO HAVE FUN WITH SOMEONE ELSE'S BODY

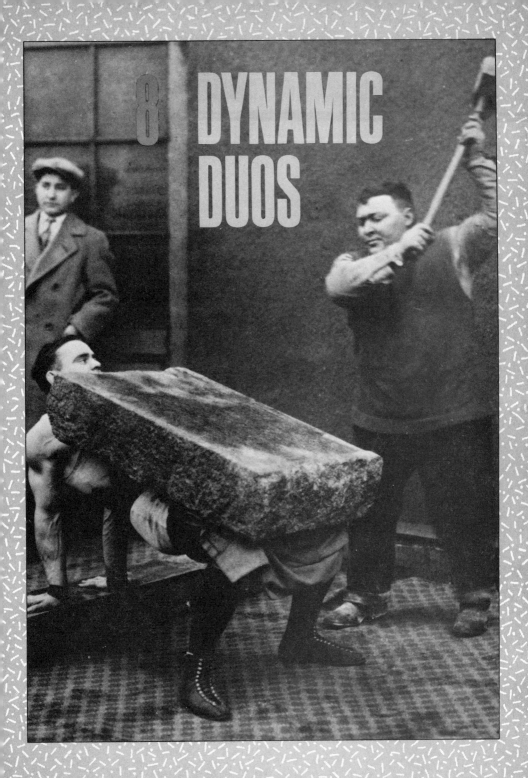

8 DYNAMIC DUOS

HIGHLY SENSITIVE AREAS

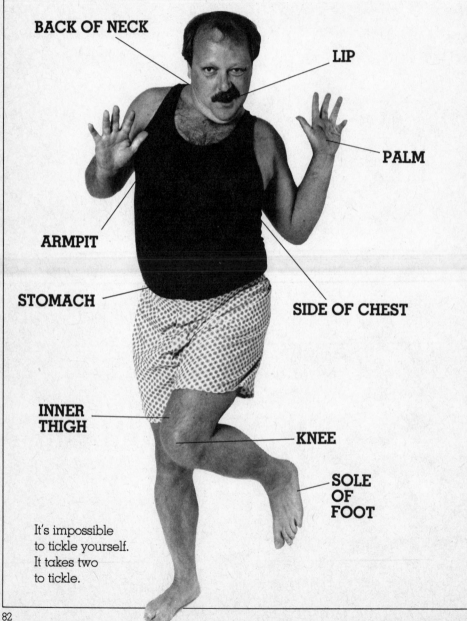

BACK OF NECK

LIP

PALM

ARMPIT

STOMACH

SIDE OF CHEST

INNER
THIGH

KNEE

SOLE
OF
FOOT

It's impossible
to tickle yourself.
It takes two
to tickle.

HOW TO FRENCH KISS

PG-13

Use your tongue.

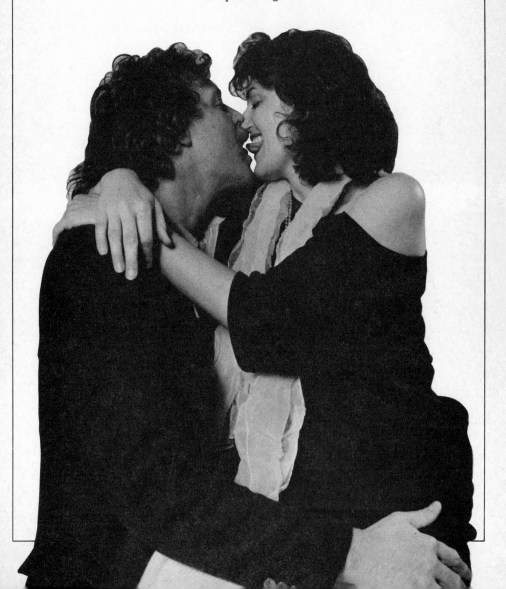

ESKIMOS AREN'T THE ONLY ONES

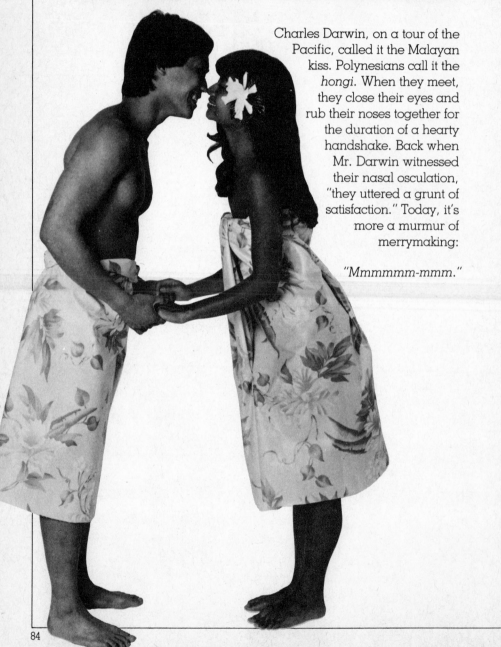

Charles Darwin, on a tour of the Pacific, called it the Malayan kiss. Polynesians call it the *hongi*. When they meet, they close their eyes and rub their noses together for the duration of a hearty handshake. Back when Mr. Darwin witnessed their nasal osculation, "they uttered a grunt of satisfaction." Today, it's more a murmur of merrymaking:

"Mmmmmm-mmm."

WHAT'S THE DEFERENCE?

In this day and age, kissing the hand is a sign of respect reserved primarily for religious leaders and royalty. With Lady Di or Bruce ("The Boss") Springsteen, you might wonder how to mind your manners. Just what does one kiss? The hand? The cheek? The feet?
With the Pope, no problem:

Kiss his ring.

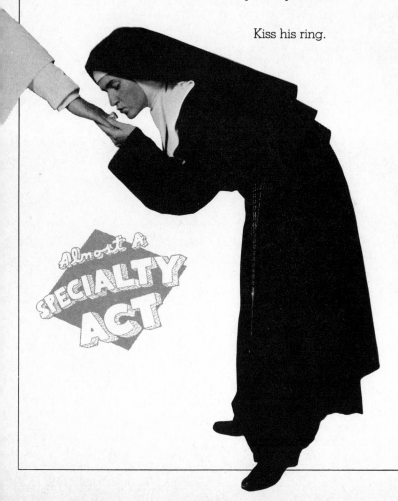

LOVE LIKE A BABY

They don't talk yet.
But babies have their own special ways
of letting you know when they can't
bear to be without you.

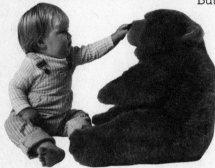

NOSE PULL

Grab his nose and repeatedly tug
on it. Don't stop until he either
(1) smiles or (2) sneezes.

LIP SMACK

Bring lips tightly together, press them
against his lips, his nose, anywhere
on his face, then hold that pose until
he gives in and kisses back.

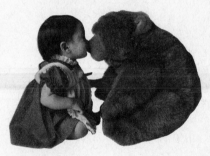

DOUBLE REVERSE

When emotions seem misdirected,
don't turn your back.
Look around — there's
always some way to
pick up his spirits.

FATHER HUG

Rest chin on his shoulder and
rub ear against his neck.
Sigh.

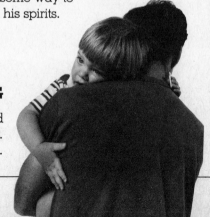

HOW TO FLIP YOUR KID

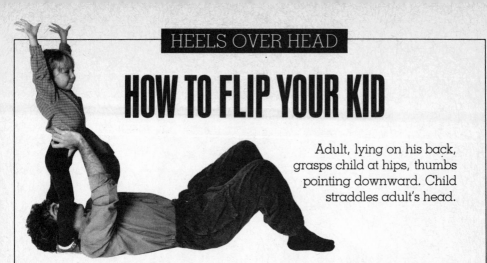

Adult, lying on his back, grasps child at hips, thumbs pointing downward. Child straddles adult's head.

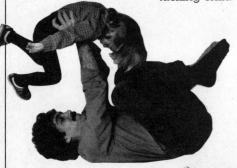

Adult, raising his feet up so shins are parallel with floor, lifts child. Child bends forward, tucking chin.

Child kicks his heels up and over as if doing a somersault. Adult guides flip, using his knees to cradle the child's shoulders and using his shins as the child's "back rest."

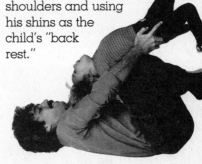

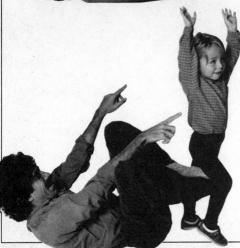

Child springs up off shins and returns to standing position. Adult laughs and glows with pride.

Ta-da!

(Warning: *Child is never satisfied with just one flip.*)

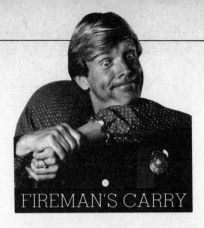

FIREMAN'S CARRY

RESCUE A DAMSEL IN DISTRESS

With damsel facing your right shoulder, **reach** between her legs and position your right hand behind her right knee.

With your left hand, **pull** her right wrist behind your neck and transfer it to your right hand. Bend your knees until her lower abdomen rests on your shoulder.

Shift your weight until you're completely centered.
Stand up.

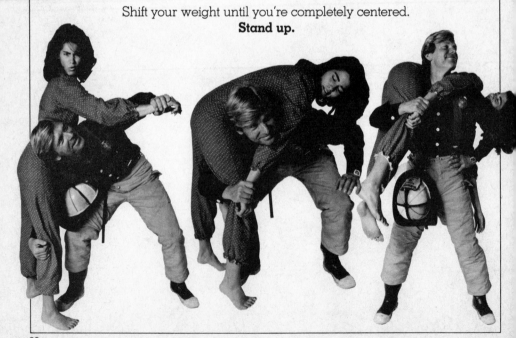

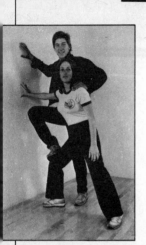

STRAIGHT FROM THE SHOULDER

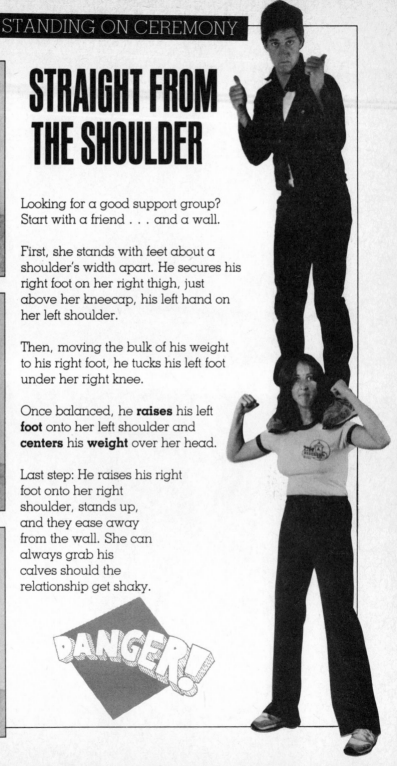

Looking for a good support group? Start with a friend . . . and a wall.

First, she stands with feet about a shoulder's width apart. He secures his right foot on her right thigh, just above her kneecap, his left hand on her left shoulder.

Then, moving the bulk of his weight to his right foot, he tucks his left foot under her right knee.

Once balanced, he **raises** his left **foot** onto her left shoulder and **centers** his **weight** over her head.

Last step: He raises his right foot onto her right shoulder, stands up, and they ease away from the wall. She can always grab his calves should the relationship get shaky.

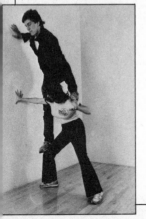

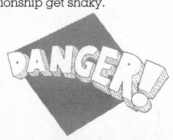

DANGER!

THE DIFFERENCE BETWEEN MEN AND WOMEN

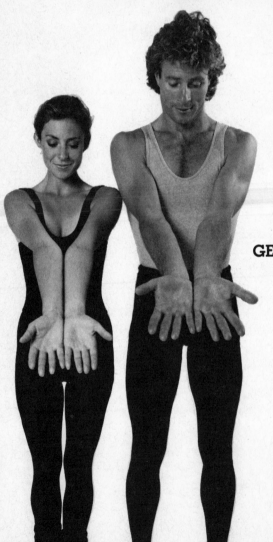

"Anatomy is destiny."
— Sigmund Freud

GEOMETRY

Extend your arms.
Women's elbows touch;
men's don't.

PHYSICS

A forearm's distance from your knee, place a tape cassette, cigarette pack, or deck of playing cards. With hands clasped behind back, try to knock over the deck with your nose.

Women can; men can't.

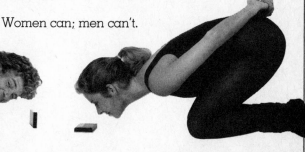

DATA PROCESSING

You're out for a night on the town. Ooops — did you step in something? Women usually study their soles over their shoulders;
men pull up their ankles.

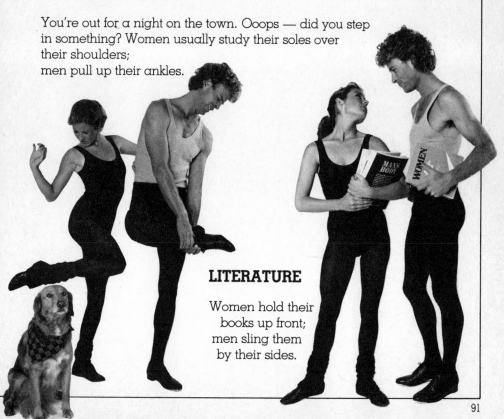

LITERATURE

Women hold their books up front; men sling them by their sides.

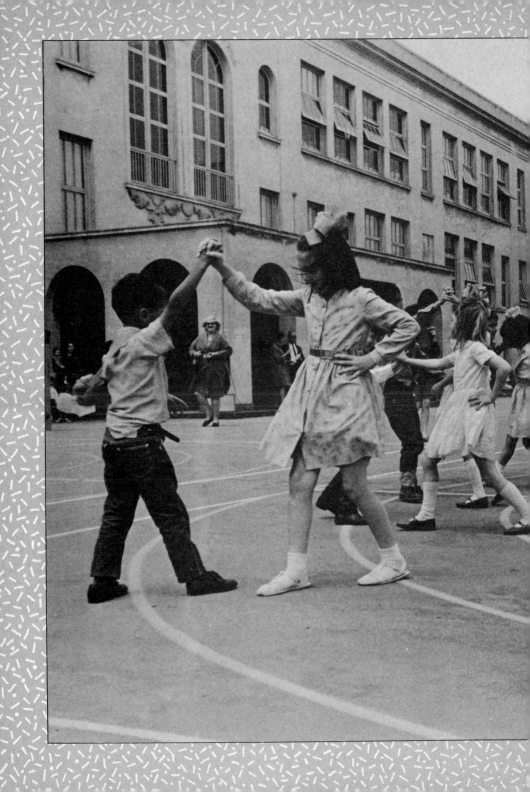

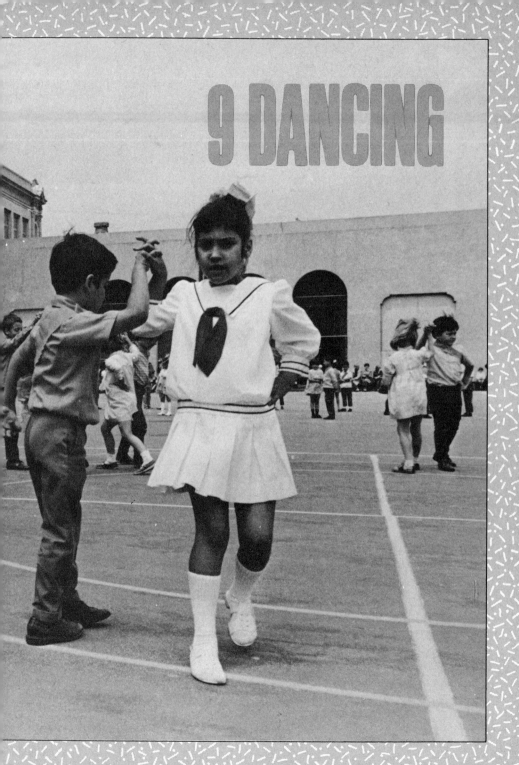

9 DANCING

HULA TO THE FIRST FOUR BARS OF THE NATIONAL ANTHEM

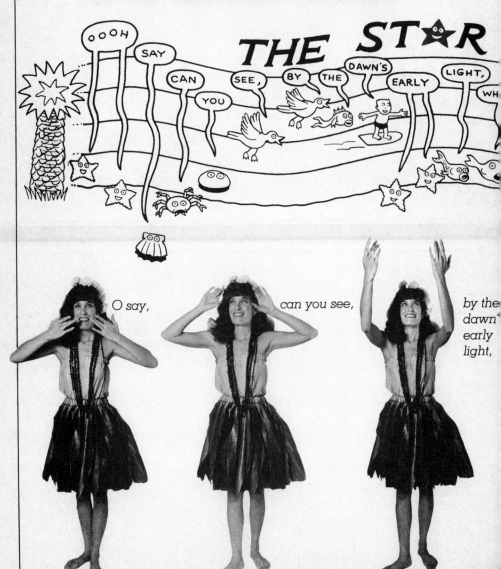

Until Captain James Cook discovered the islands in 1778, Hawaii was populated just with Hawaiians. They had no written language, just an expressive vocabulary full of flowing vowels and a kind of sign language full of flowing gestures. There are hundreds of graceful, soft, sensuous movements to the hula. Interpretation of a song is left up to the individual performer, and every Hawaiian dancer has her (or his) own style. Anything goes, as long as you go with the flow.

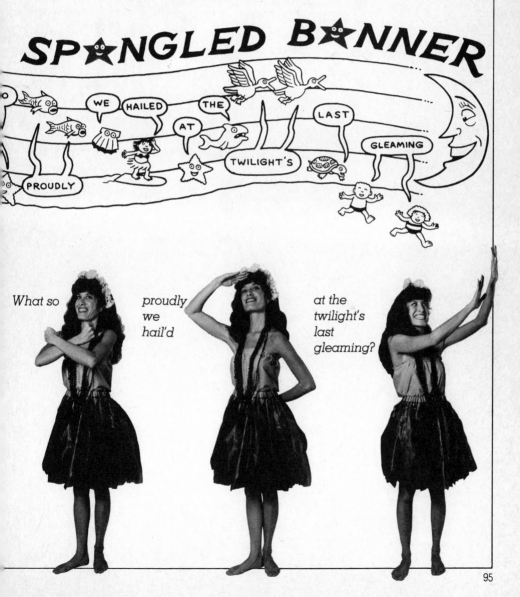

HOW TO BE THE VERY WEST YOU CAN BE

Deep in the heart of Texas, we got us a perdy little dance, but we do it in a big way. The two-step likes lots of room. Ya'll needn't turn 'round. Ya'll needn't change direction. Ya'll just parade in a circle, the cowboy leadin' with his left, the cowgirl backsteppin' with her right. Two slow steps then, sure 'nough, two quick ones. Keep ya'll's back straight and ya'll's weight on the balls of ya'll's feet. And have a mighty good time, ya hear?

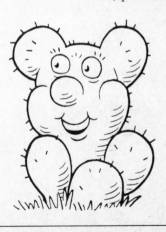

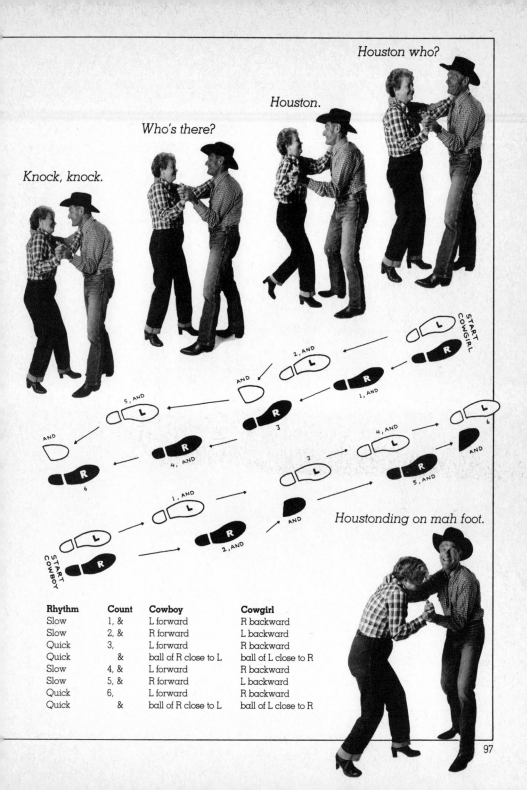

Knock, knock.

Who's there?

Houston.

Houston who?

Houstonding on mah foot.

Rhythm	Count	Cowboy	Cowgirl
Slow	1, &	L forward	R backward
Slow	2, &	R forward	L backward
Quick	3,	L forward	R backward
Quick	&	ball of R close to L	ball of L close to R
Slow	4, &	L forward	R backward
Slow	5, &	R forward	L backward
Quick	6,	L forward	R backward
Quick	&	ball of R close to L	ball of L close to R

HOW TO WALTZ

The waltz today is the same as it was 200 years ago in Bavaria: forward (or backward), sideways, then close — elegantly executed in ¾ time.

Practice the box step. If you can glide through a box step and add a turn, you can waltz. It's as easy as ONE-two-three, ONE-two-three.

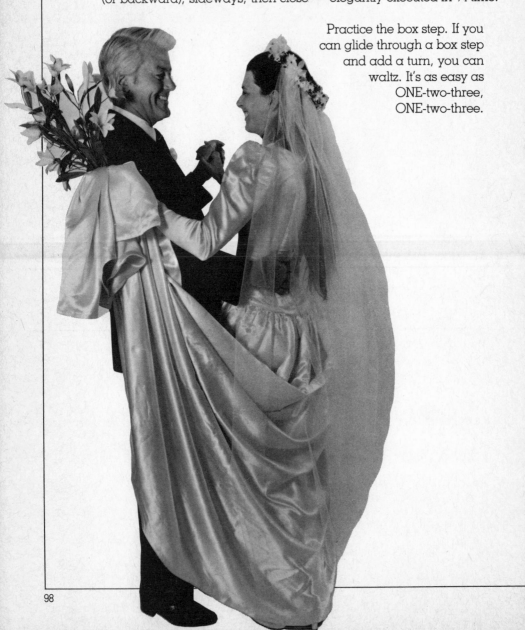

The Left Box Step*

Count	Gentleman	Lady
1	L forward	R backward
2	R sideways	L sideways
3	L close to R	R close to L
4	R backward	L forward
5	L sideways	R sideways
6	R close to L	L close to R

For right box step, gentleman starts L backward, lady starts R forward.

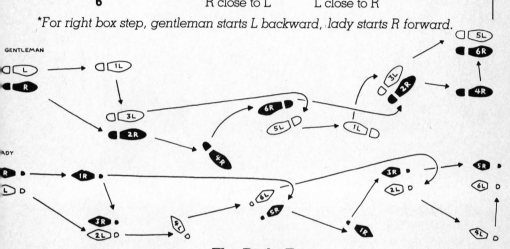

The Right Turn

Count	Gentleman	Lady	
1	L forward	R backward	
2	R sideways	L sideways	
3	L close to R	R close to L	
4	R forward	L backward	Turn right to face in opposite direction.
5	L sideways	R sideways	
6	R close to L	L close to R	
1	L backward	R forward	
2	R sideways	L sideways	
3	L close to R	R close to L	
4	R forward	L backward	Turn right to face in original direction.
5	L sideways	R sideways	
6	R close to L	L close to R	

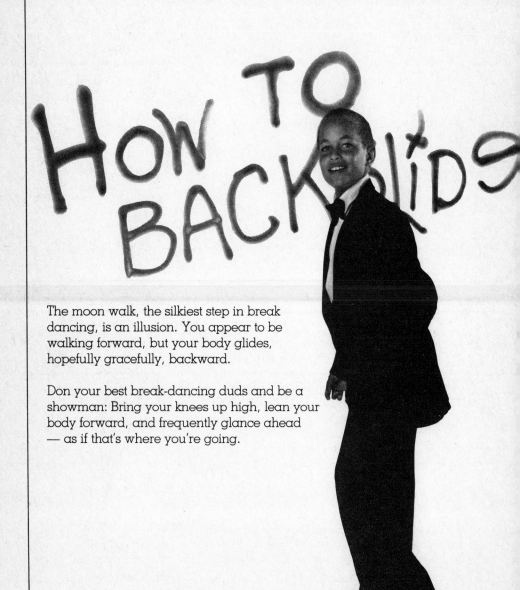

HOW TO BACKSLIDE

The moon walk, the silkiest step in break dancing, is an illusion. You appear to be walking forward, but your body glides, hopefully gracefully, backward.

Don your best break-dancing duds and be a showman: Bring your knees up high, lean your body forward, and frequently glance ahead — as if that's where you're going.

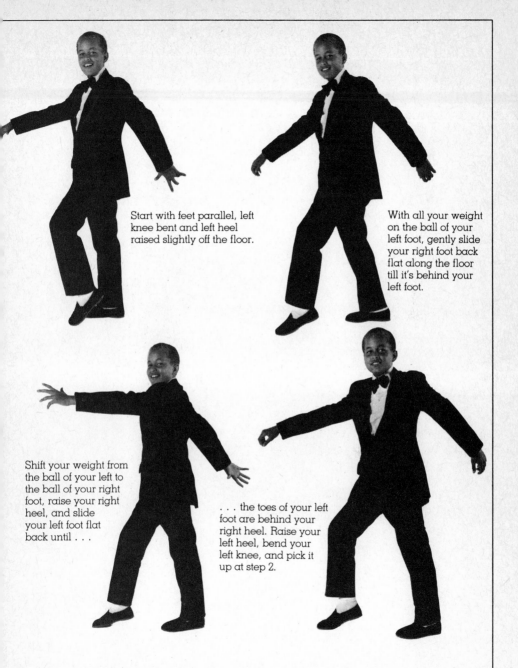

Start with feet parallel, left knee bent and left heel raised slightly off the floor.

With all your weight on the ball of your left foot, gently slide your right foot back flat along the floor till it's behind your left foot.

Shift your weight from the ball of your left to the ball of your right foot, raise your right heel, and slide your left foot flat back until . . .

. . . the toes of your left foot are behind your right heel. Raise your left heel, bend your left knee, and pick it up at step 2.

Practice in front of a store window or a long, uninterrupted mirror.

THE FIVE BASIC BALLET POSITIONS

Support yourself by gripping the back of a chair, a dresser or, should one be available, a barre. Distribute your weight evenly on both feet. Keep your shoulders down and your back straight. Raise your diaphragm and ribs. Tighten your stomach and buttocks muscles. Put your best foot forward and follow the numbers:

1. Keeping heels together, rotate your toes out to the side. For safety's sake, be sure to turn the entire leg out from the hip.

2. Assume the first position. Slide your feet apart. The gap between the heels should be equal to the length of your own foot.

3. Assume the second position. Bring the heel of your front foot to the instep of your back foot. Try not to roll the foot, but keep your soles firmly on the floor.

4. Assume the third position. With toes pointing out and your feet as parallel as possible, move your front foot forward till it's about a foot's length in front of your back toes.

5. Assume the fourth position. Move your front foot back till its heel touches the toes of the back foot and its toes touch the heel of the back foot. The fifth position is the most frequently used and certainly the most difficult.

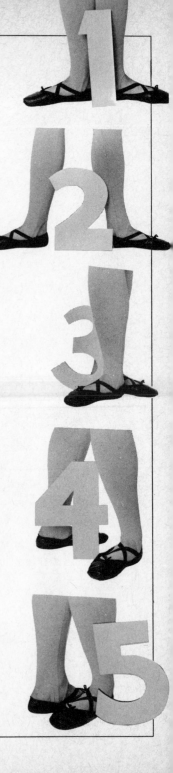

10 GROUP DYNAMICS

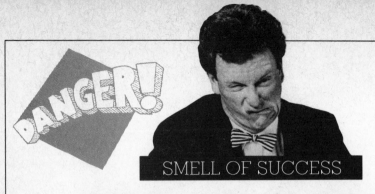

SMELL OF SUCCESS

HOW TO STAND ON A FACE

"In those days we had faces." — Gloria Swanson

Don't try this trick at home. Don't even try it at someone else's home. It requires strong lifting muscles in the hands and arms. It requires faces that can be stepped on. Don't try this trick. It can be extremely painful and is potentially hazardous to the future of your children. Don't even think about trying it.

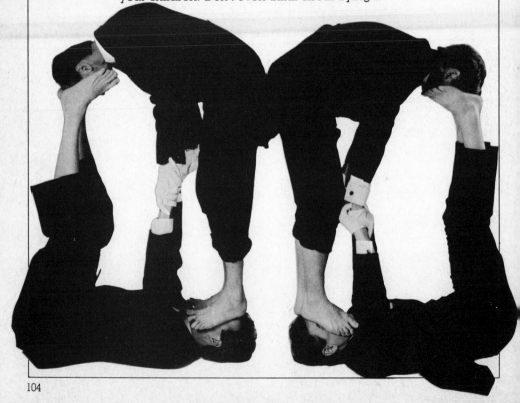

STUNTS AND STAGE FIGHTS

Act out your anger. Mash 'em, bash 'em, thrash 'em, trash 'em, slash 'em, and smash 'em till they come crashing down. Then, for good measure, kick 'em where it hurts.

Well, not really. You just **pretend.**

Practice carefully — in slow motion — with the utmost concern for the body you are pretending to bruise. Judge your distance, accentuate the histrionics and, to be on the safe side, have your buddy sign a waiver against damages.

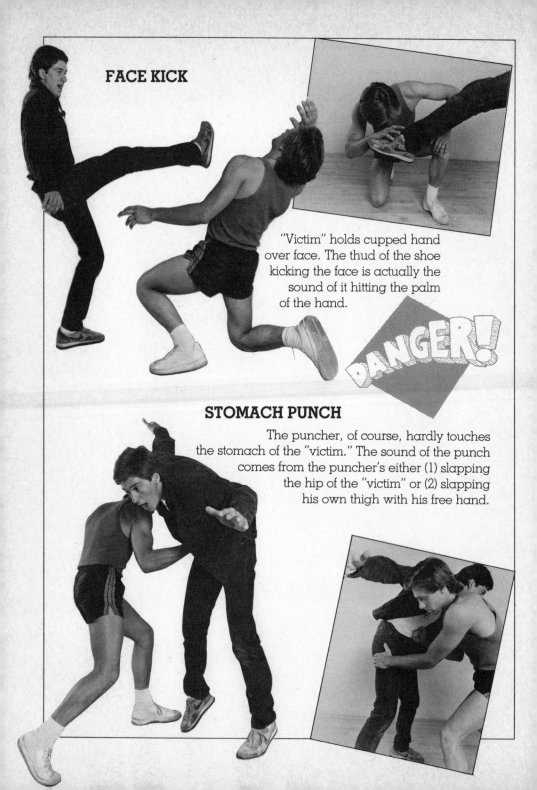

FACE KICK

"Victim" holds cupped hand over face. The thud of the shoe kicking the face is actually the sound of it hitting the palm of the hand.

DANGER!

STOMACH PUNCH

The puncher, of course, hardly touches the stomach of the "victim." The sound of the punch comes from the puncher's either (1) slapping the hip of the "victim" or (2) slapping his own thigh with his free hand.

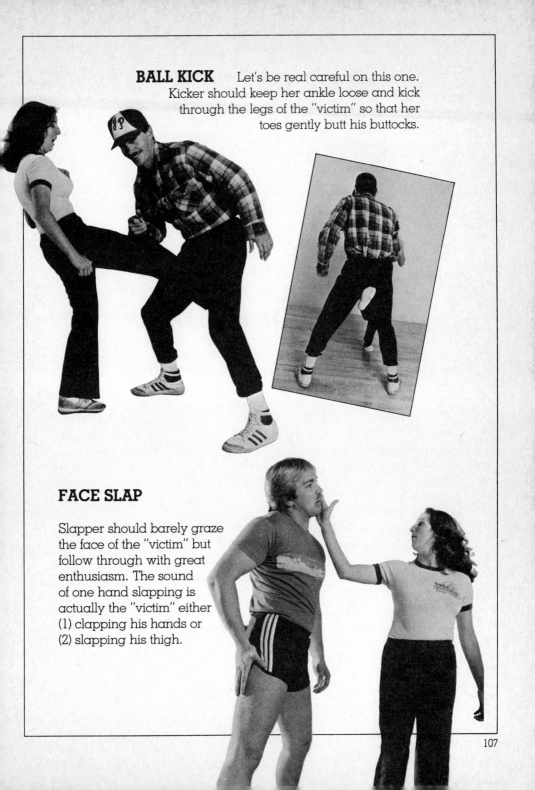

BALL KICK   Let's be real careful on this one. Kicker should keep her ankle loose and kick through the legs of the "victim" so that her toes gently butt his buttocks.

FACE SLAP

Slapper should barely graze the face of the "victim" but follow through with great enthusiasm. The sound of one hand slapping is actually the "victim" either (1) clapping his hands or (2) slapping his thigh.

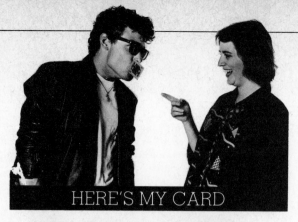

THE PARTY SUCKS— LET'S BLOW THIS SCENE

Forget "Pass the Orange" and "Post Office." The most popular getting-to-know-you game around is "Suck and Blow," a hit more for its moniker than for the way the game is played, viz.:

Two lines of boy-girl-boy-girl compete. The first boy in each line sucks a card to his lips (any business or credit card will do; yuppies prefer to use an American Express card). He then tries to pass it to the girl behind him without either of them using hands. How? She "kisses" the card and also **sucks** while he simultaneously stops sucking and **blows.** Then she, still inhaling, must pass the card to the boy behind her. First group to pass the card down the line wins the game.

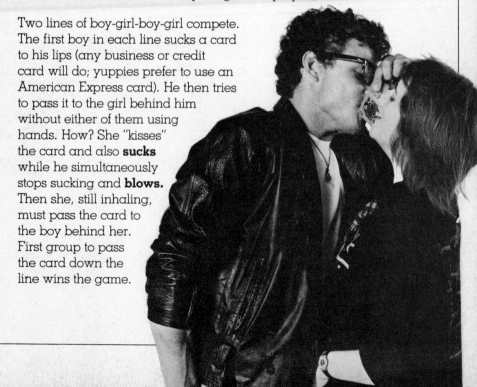

PASS THE PERSON, PLEASE

"Forget being the bright, successful you — simply be a body."
— Helen Gurley Brown

Pick a victim.

Everybody else gets down and gets funky, forming two parallel
rows, buttocks in abutment, legs in the air.
The victim falls aboard and is passed down the line.
The first person to drop the passee becomes the next person
to be passed, please.

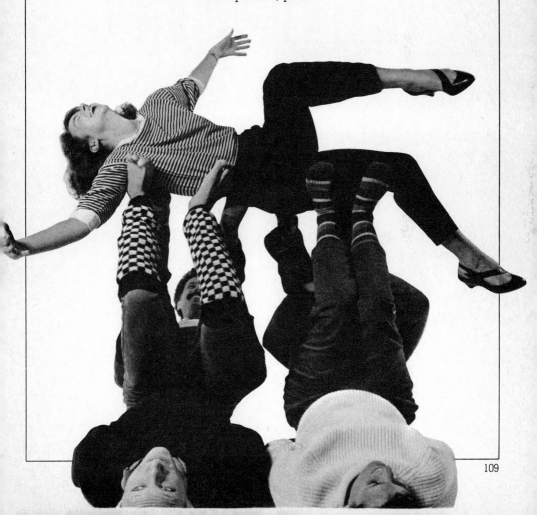

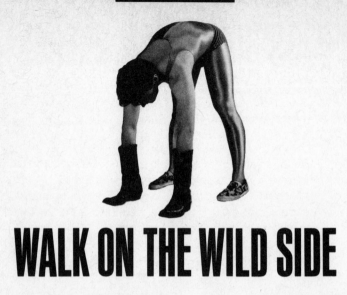

WALK ON THE WILD SIDE

The last segment of the centipede (known to the others as "our tail") **bends** over so his feet and hands are flat on the floor, stable and sturdy. The second segment crouches next to the tail and sidles onto the tail's back. He rests his hands in front of the tail's, tucks his knees around the tail's pelvic area, and locks his ankles together. Everybody **mounts** in the same fashion, until all the segments are present and accounted for.

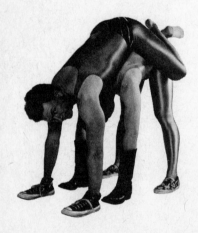

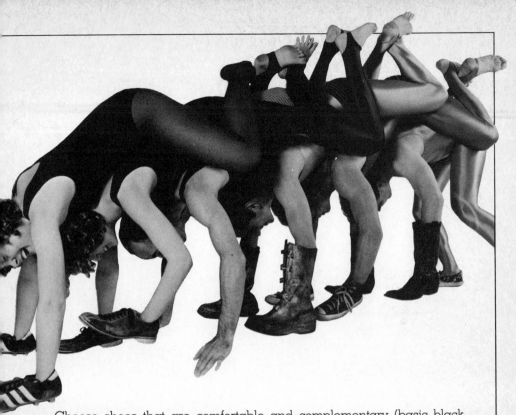

Choose shoes that are comfortable and complementary (basic black goes with everything). When all segments are connected and resting securely, sound off and pick up shoes in unison. Step in place: left, right, left. Once there's some semblance of Segment Coordination, move 'em on out. Forward, **crawl.**

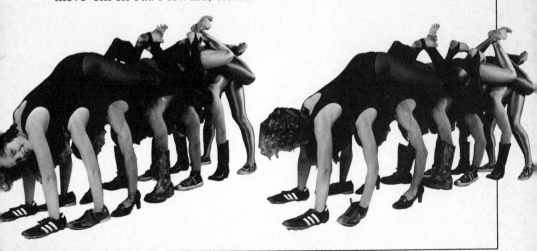

THE CABLE CAR THAT COULD

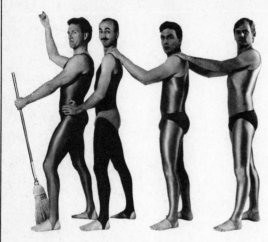

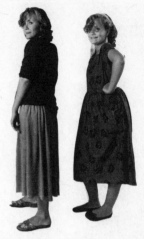

Once upon a time, not so long ago, a cable car waited patiently for passengers to climb inside.

Along came the twins, tourists they were, each with a ticket to ride.

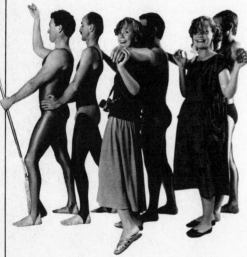

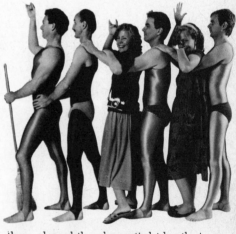

They opened the doors, and climbed aboard,

then closed the doors tight by their sides. Hold on, they did. Hold tight, they did. "Let's head for the hills," they cried.

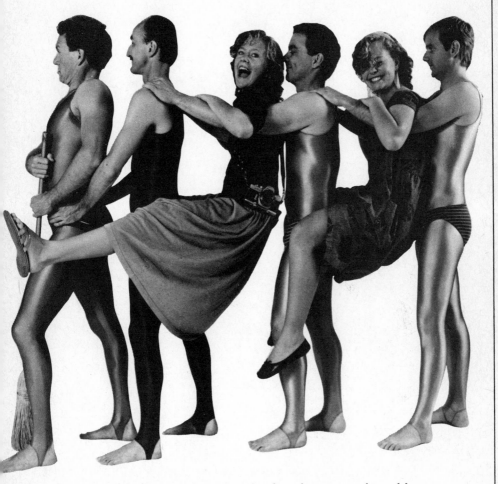

They kicked up their heels and sat back in their seats; the cable car started to fly. The twins yelled, "What a thrill" as they zoomed up the hill, while the cable car took it in stride. Of course.

SIGN LANGUAGE

CHARADES

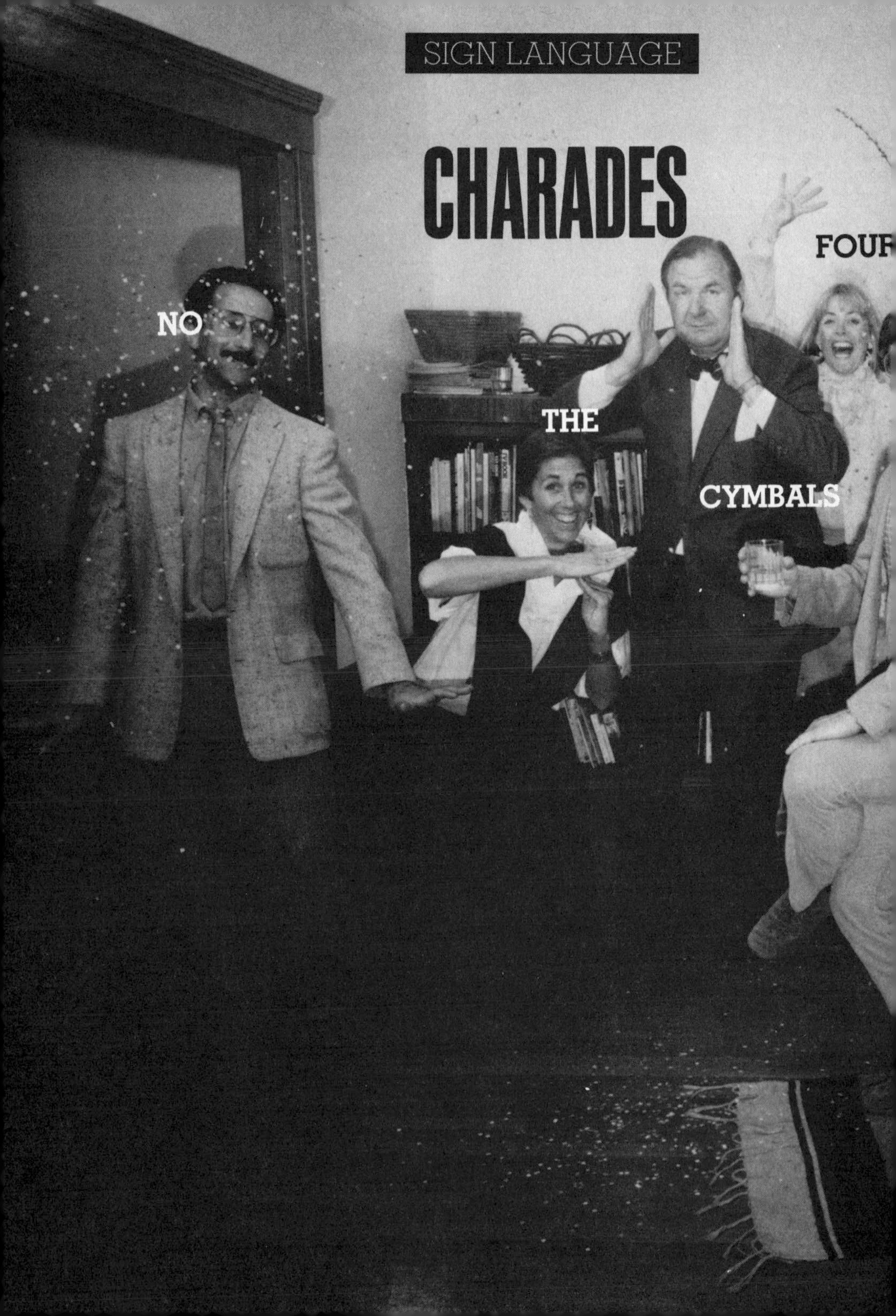

NO

THE

CYMBALS

FOUR

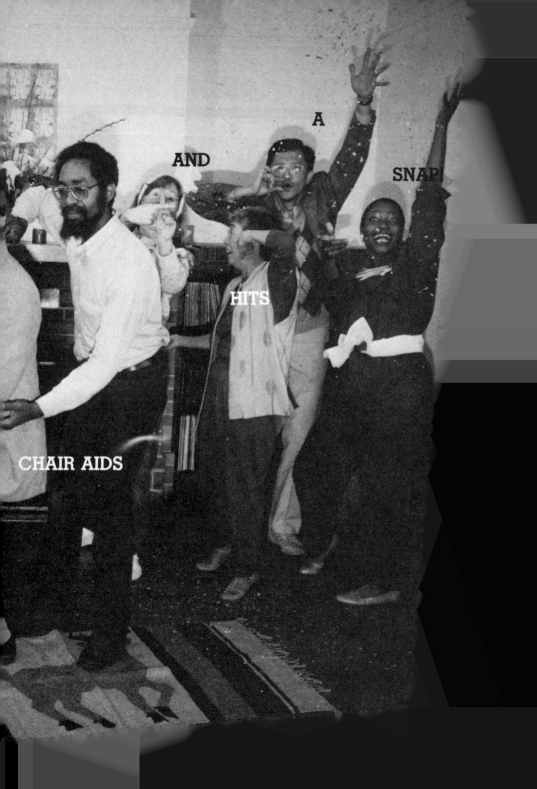

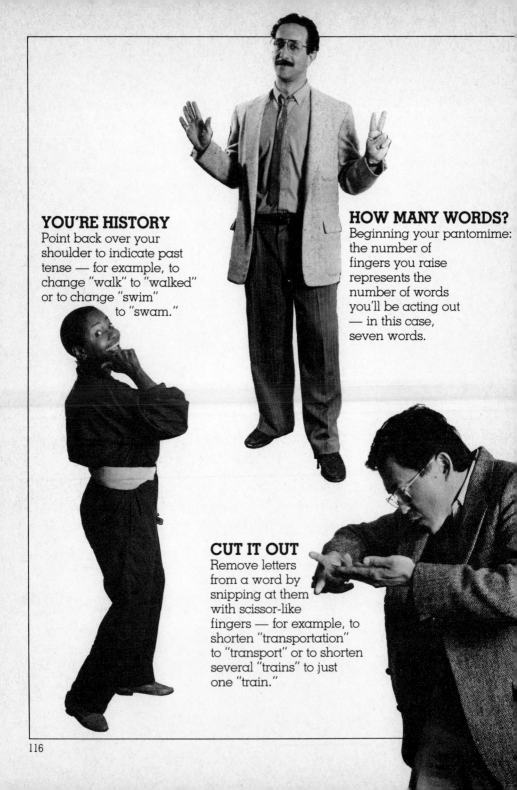

YOU'RE HISTORY
Point back over your shoulder to indicate past tense — for example, to change "walk" to "walked" or to change "swim" to "swam."

HOW MANY WORDS?
Beginning your pantomime: the number of fingers you raise represents the number of words you'll be acting out — in this case, seven words.

CUT IT OUT
Remove letters from a word by snipping at them with scissor-like fingers — for example, to shorten "transportation" to "transport" or to shorten several "trains" to just one "train."

ON THE BUTTON

When someone in your audience shouts out the correct word or phrase, immediately point to him or her and touch your other finger to your nose.

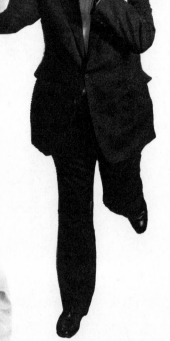

Around

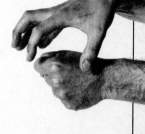

OKAY, LET'S TAKE IT SYLLABLE BY SYLLABLE

Place fingers of right hand on left forearm to indicate number of syllables — in this case, a two-syllable word.

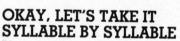

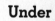

Under

Over

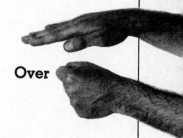

THE WHOLE IDEA

When you need several actions to portray a single word, first signal the Whole Idea. For example, for "family," first hold your arms in a big circle, then you can act out the family members — mommy, baby, daddy, etc.

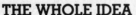

SOUNDS LIKE

If a word is hard to mime, try one that rhymes with it. For example, for "missing," act out "kissing" and, when your audience hits it on the button, tug your ear lobe and have them guess words that sound like "kissing."

STREEEETCH IT OUT

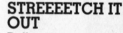

Pull apart imaginary taffy when you want to change verb tenses or add "ing" endings, plurals, or extra letters — for example, changing "grove" to "groove."

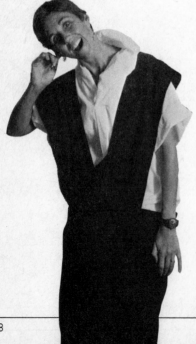

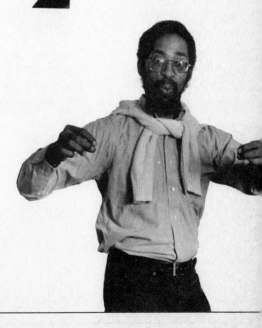

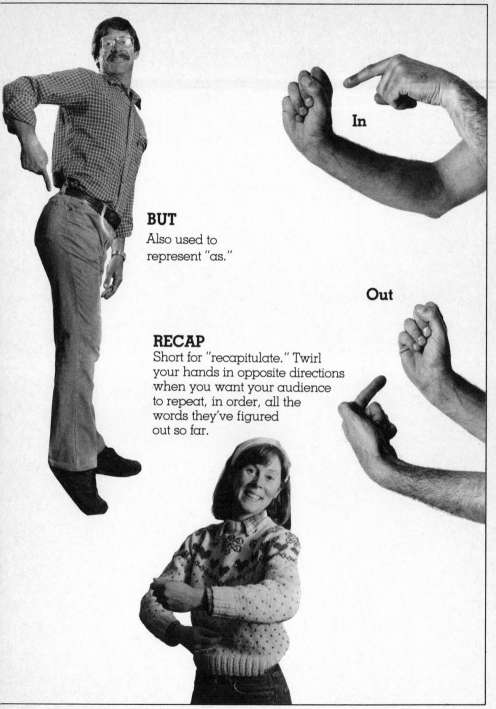

In

BUT
Also used to
represent "as."

Out

RECAP
Short for "recapitulate." Twirl
your hands in opposite directions
when you want your audience
to repeat, in order, all the
words they've figured
out so far.

HOW TO IMPERSONATE THE GOLDEN GATE BRIDGE

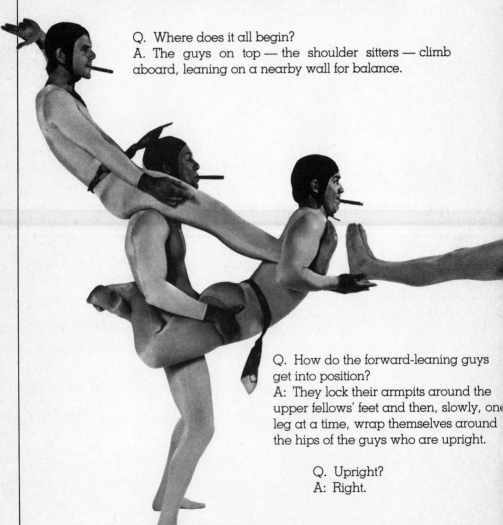

Q. Where does it all begin?
A. The guys on top — the shoulder sitters — climb aboard, leaning on a nearby wall for balance.

Q. How do the forward-leaning guys get into position?
A: They lock their armpits around the upper fellows' feet and then, slowly, one leg at a time, wrap themselves around the hips of the guys who are upright.

Q. Upright?
A: Right.

Q: How long can they stay there like that? Forever?
A: As long as they remain balanced.

Q: What are they smoking cigars for?
A: Fog.

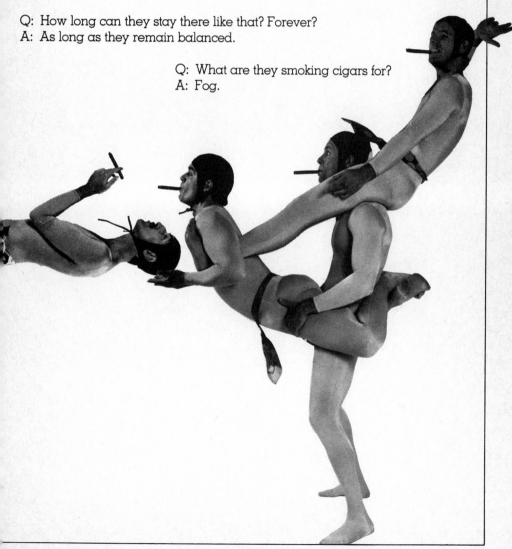

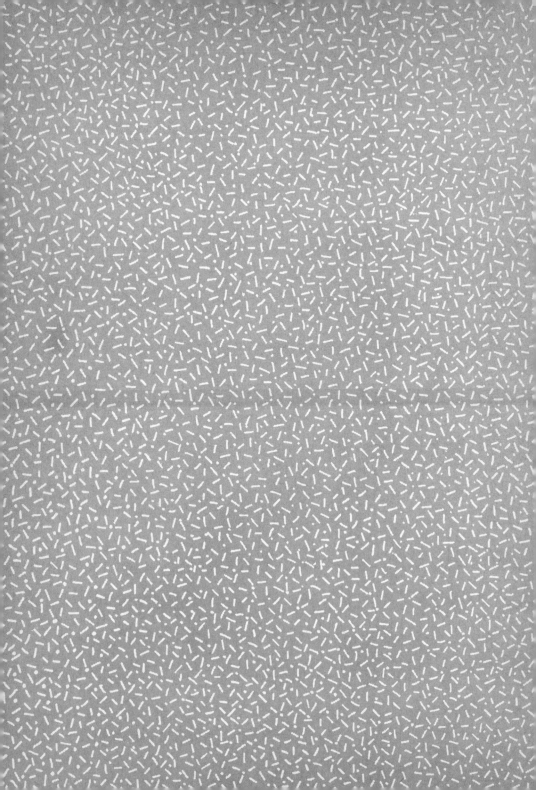

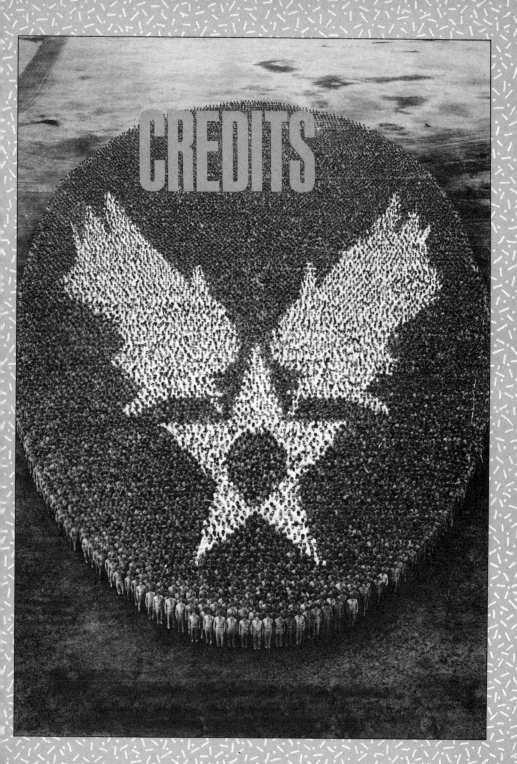

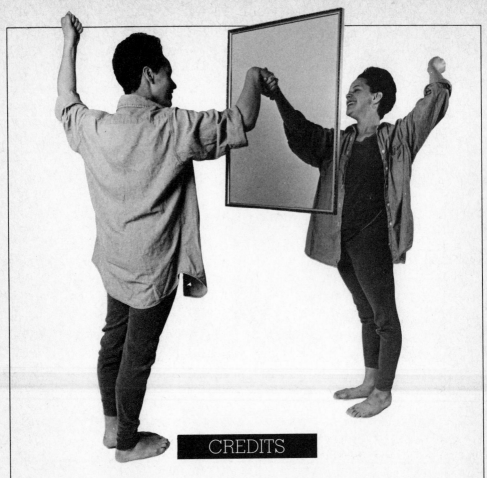

CREDITS

We'd like to thank our models for their behavior:

Michael Aczon, 84
Jules Bachus, 49
Clayton Bailey, 32
Betty and Warren Boggess, 98–99
Noriko Bridges, 115, 118
Dick Bright, 19, 35
Victoria Bugarin, 84
Eddie Cantor, 21
Sterling Christiansan, 90–91
Rachel Carroll, 108
Shana Carroll, 36–37
Bruce Charonnat, 41

Devon Chatley, 86
Norman Chun, 115–117
Jill Clarke, 94–95
Paul Cohen, 114, 116
Margaret Connell, 48
Fred Crowe, 108
Lowell Darling, 18, 78–79
Simone Davalos, 19, 22
Stuart Drake, 88, 105–106
Lloyd Ehrenberg, 19, 109
Greg Ferrando, 105–106
Fratelli Bologna

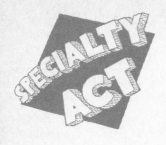

SPECIAL THANKS

To **Ellen Weber,** chalkboard coordinator, for her line-by-line coaching, her colorful commentary, and her willingness to play hard and play dirty; to **Nancy Hayes,** our head scout, our link with the players, a good sport and a real reconnoiterer; to **Denise Austin,** for letting us stretch the truth to "Tone Up at the Terminals"; to **Janet Tallman,** for assisting during the kick-off; to **Julie Nishino** and to **Geri Handa,** for carrying the ball; to **Travis Amos** and to **Sayre van Young** for researching the field; to **Jim Mayer,** for providing fast breaks and warm huddles; to **Gerard Van der Leun,** our head coach at Houghton Mifflin, our own private pep rally, a place-kicker who can spot an errant projectile faster than you can say Gerard Van der Leun; and to Captain Hook, Vincent van Gogh, Marie Antoinette, Long John Silver, and all those marvelous men and women who gave a part of themselves that this book might live.

HEY!

Have you heard of any good gags?
Have you got a trick up your sleeve?
One that you're willing to share with strangers?
Great!

Please send your special act to:

THE BOD SQUAD

Houghton Mifflin Company
Two Park Street
Boston, Massachusetts 02108

We're all ears.

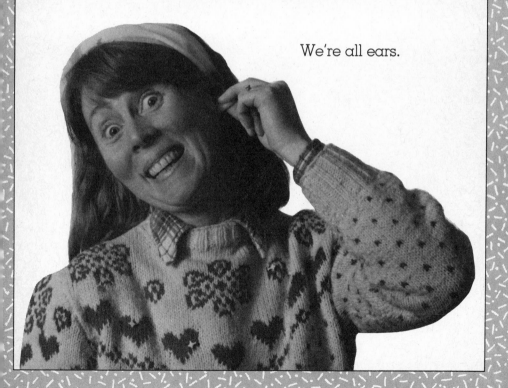

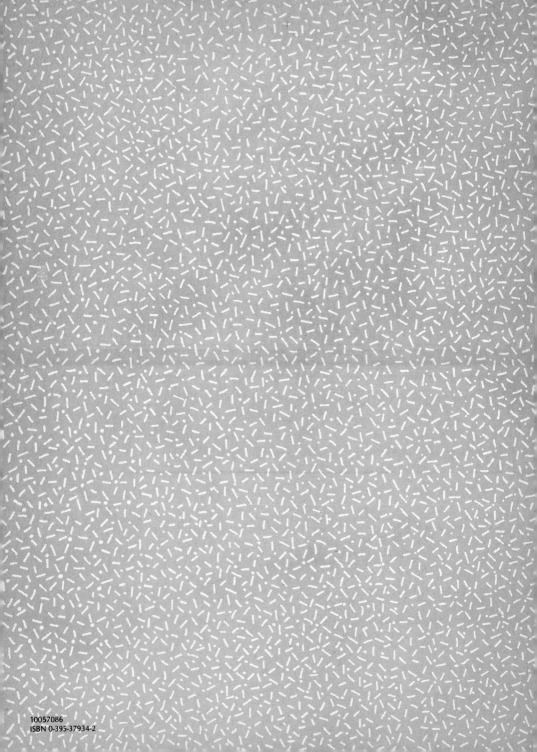

10057086
ISBN 0-395-37934-2